Rossen Dimov

Pitfalls and complications of laparoscopic cholecystectomy

Rossen Dimov

Pitfalls and complications of laparoscopic cholecystectomy

LAP LAMBERT Academic Publishing

Impressum / Imprint

Bibliografische Information der Deutschen Nationalbibliothek: Die Deutsche Nationalbibliothek verzeichnet diese Publikation in der Deutschen Nationalbibliografie; detaillierte bibliografische Daten sind im Internet über http://dnb.d-nb.de abrufbar.

Alle in diesem Buch genannten Marken und Produktnamen unterliegen warenzeichen-, marken- oder patentrechtlichem Schutz bzw. sind Warenzeichen oder eingetragene Warenzeichen der jeweiligen Inhaber. Die Wiedergabe von Marken, Produktnamen, Gebrauchsnamen, Handelsnamen, Warenbezeichnungen u.s.w. in diesem Werk berechtigt auch ohne besondere Kennzeichnung nicht zu der Annahme, dass solche Namen im Sinne der Warenzeichen- und Markenschutzgesetzgebung als frei zu betrachten wären und daher von jedermann benutzt werden dürften.

Bibliographic information published by the Deutsche Nationalbibliothek: The Deutsche Nationalbibliothek lists this publication in the Deutsche Nationalbibliografie; detailed bibliographic data are available in the Internet at http://dnb.d-nb.de.

Any brand names and product names mentioned in this book are subject to trademark, brand or patent protection and are trademarks or registered trademarks of their respective holders. The use of brand names, product names, common names, trade names, product descriptions etc. even without a particular marking in this works is in no way to be construed to mean that such names may be regarded as unrestricted in respect of trademark and brand protection legislation and could thus be used by anyone.

Coverbild / Cover image: www.ingimage.com

Verlag / Publisher:
LAP LAMBERT Academic Publishing
ist ein Imprint der / is a trademark of
OmniScriptum GmbH & Co. KG
Heinrich-Böcking-Str. 6-8, 66121 Saarbrücken, Deutschland / Germany
Email: info@lap-publishing.com

Herstellung: siehe letzte Seite /
Printed at: see last page
ISBN: 978-3-659-58040-6

Copyright © 2014 OmniScriptum GmbH & Co. KG
Alle Rechte vorbehalten. / All rights reserved. Saarbrücken 2014

Rossen Stoyanov Dimov

Danger points, pitfalls and complications in laparoscopic cholecystectomy

General Surgery Clinic, University Hospital "Kaspela" - Ltd. Plovdiv. Department of Surgery, Medical University of Plovdiv.

Plovdiv

2013

Author: Associate Professor Rosen Stoyanov Dimov, MD, Ph. D.
Artist-illustrator: Kirila Georgieva

Contents

Introduction

In the last decade laparoscopy has become the gold standard in the implementation of the majority of procedures in the abdominal cavity. Despite standardized protocols for education and training, practical schooling for all surgeons starts and for the most part continues with the implementation of laparoscopic cholecystectomy. Since the dawn of its implementation to the present time it has become a "best seller", the most often practiced laparoscopic procedure in general surgery. All innovations in the improvement of laparoscopy as the technique of single-port surgery and NOTES technology have made their first steps with the performance of cholecystectomy. Huge in quantity and quality information has been accumulated on how to perform the operation. And amid this rapid development as "a thorn in the Achilles' heel "possible errors, threats and complications of laparoscopic cholecystectomy remain, which invariably accompany each of us in the constant path of improvement. Unfortunately, neither modern technologies, nor team work principle have resulted in the elimination of Intraoperative complications. Their share remains at approximately the same range for the last five years. Learning and self-perfection oriented behaviour can protect to a large extent by the bitterness of "failure" and the complicated treatment of iatrogenic influenced patients. In this aspect, I consider right a sentence that crystallized during the accumulation of my personal experience in laparoscopic surgery. It reads: "A surgeon is ready to perform alone an operational procedure, only when he is ready to meet and adequately treat potential complications." I hope that this practice-oriented book will help the majority of my colleagues to avoid worries and sleepless nights that are part of the professional path of each of us.

I would be grateful for any feedback, guidelines or comments that would enrich or improve the content of this book.

The author

Chapter one

Review and classification of complications in laparoscopic cholecystectomy

I.   Overview

After categorical proof of the undoubted efficiency of laparoscopic cholecystectomy over open surgery, main emphasis has been placed on patient safety. In this respect numerous studies have been published over the years on mortality and complications of laparoscopic procedures. Summative data analysis shows significantly lowered mortality - from 0.0% to 0.1% compared with the 1.5% to 2% in open surgery. /1, 6/ Regarding complications, data show a relative balance between the two surgical techniques, the total share being 1% -5.1%, with severe (life-threatening) complications in 0.7% -2%, and minor complications in up to 4% of cases. /1,2,6/ There is only one small difference without statistical reliability concerning injury of the common bile duct - 1.5% for laparoscopic surgery and 0.9% for open surgery./6,17/ In the early years of introduction of the operative technique, the lower proportion of deaths and serious complications in laparoscopic cholecystectomy was explained by many surgeons with strict indications for the operation. As we now know, indications and contraindications underwent significant changes over time in order to reach the present stage in practically no contraindications for this operating technique.

Studies in the last five years reaffirm the significantly lower mortality and the equivalent share of complications compared with the open technique. In this aspect, laparoscopic cholecystectomy is a long-established "gold" standard for the surgical treatment of gallbladder diseases and also a procedure, launching the training of surgeons in highly specialized activities in laparoscopic surgery.

II.   Classification of complications

In order to study and effectively prevent complications of laparoscopic cholecystectomy, they need to be systematized and classified according to specific criteria. Available literature presents   different classifications depending on the complications themselves or the criteria of systematizing. I apply our simplified classification where general criteria are the different stages of operational methodology. For clarification I have to mention that this classification refers to and reflects our experience in performing the standard laparoscopic procedure and single port cholecystectomy (SILS), which we practice since 2002. We have no experience and do not relate this text to cholecystectomy through a natural orifice (NOTES).

1. **Complications associated with the creation of pneumoperitoneum and placement of trocars and ports of the abdominal wall**

1.1 Vascular injuries
1.2 Injuries to internal organs
1.3 Extraperitoneal insufflation

2. **Complications associated with surgical techniques**

2.1 Injuries to the abdominal organs
2.2 Bleeding in the operative field
2.3 Injuries to the bile ducts
2.4 Injuries to the diaphragm and pleura
2.5 Obstruction of bile duct by residual or passed gallstones
2.6 Spilling of gallstones into the peritoneal cavity
2.7 Suppuration of surgical wound
2.8 Formation of postoperative hernia

We believe that the classification provided allows for detailed examination of each group of complications with emphasis on the threats, difficulties and ways to prevent them. In what follows we will examine in detail every aspect of the various groups of complications.

Chapter two

Specific information

I. Complications associated with the creation of pneumoperitoneum and insertion of trocars and ports of the abdominal wall

As known, there are two basic methods to create enough space in the peritoneal cavity for clear vision in instrumentation and manipulations on the gallbladder. One of them is the so-called lifting method in which the anterior abdominal wall is tracted upward by means of retractors. This method is extremely rare and is not applied in general practice. Widely used is the method of creation of pneumoperitoneum with carbon dioxide to a pressure of 12-13 mm Hg which allows a clear view of all compartments of the peritoneal cavity, and an excellent opportunity to use various instruments. There is definite proof that these pressures do not result in the development of compartment syndrome and allow safe work for hours on end. In this sense, the method is globally accepted and we will look into the threats and complications associated with its application.

1. Complications associated with the insertion of the Veress needle and the first trocar

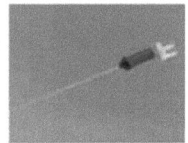

Figure 1 – Veress needle

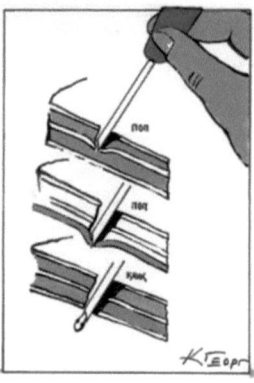

Figure 2 – Passing the needle through the layers of the abdominal wall

The needle is usually inserted in the area immediately above or below the umbilicus. The characteristic movement when passing through the layers of the abdominal wall leads to a feeling of having passed through two obstacles, and two "clicks" are heard upon penetration into the peritoneal cavity. Figure 2

Correct insertion of the needle is the most important first step towards creating a safe pneumoperitoneum. The patient is placed in slight Trendelenburg position. Upward traction of the abdominal wall is performed. We use a method of traction in which the operator grips the abdominal wall below the navel with the left hand, and the assistant lifts the abdominal wall above the umbilicus with his left hand. Puncture site is just above the navel, due to the lack of blood vessels in the abdominal wall in this area, and the fact that the parietal peritoneum is firmly adherent to the fascia of the linea alba. The angle of insertion of the needle is about 45 degrees to the horizontal line and the tip pointing towards the pelvis. Figure 3

Figure 3 – Angle of orientation of the needle

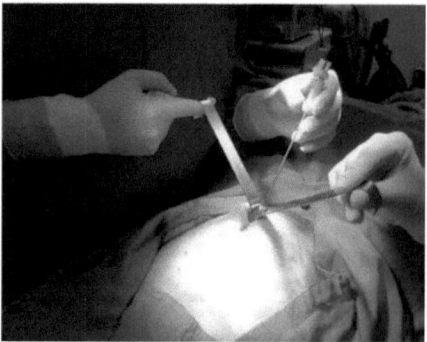

Thus the probability of the major blood vessels injury is reduced. Next step is the confirmation of the intraperitoneal location of the needle. This could be done in two ways. The first test used is free passage of a drop of saline through the needle into the peritoneal cavity. 10 cc syringe with 5 ml of physiological saline solution is connected with Veress needle and aspiration of I ml is done. If there is no aspirated blood, intestinal contents or any other liquid, the assistant raises the abdominal wall and 2-3 drops of solution are dropped into the needle. When the needle is properly positioned, the drops should move freely. Figures 4 и 5

Figure 4 – Aspiration

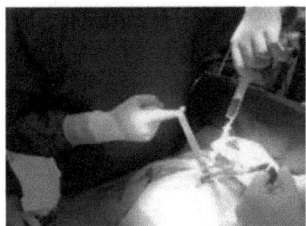

Figure 5 – Administration of saline solution

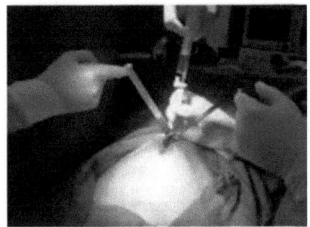

The second follow-up test is to connect the needle connector to the automatic insufflator. If the reading is 0 or negative pressure of -1, -2 mm Hg, it is a sure sign that the needle tip is inside the free peritoneal cavity. The third and last test is the monitoring of pressure in the peritoneal cavity during insufflation, which in the initial stages should remain low and gradually increase to the selected desired value. Typically, to reach a value of 10-12 mm Hg, around 4-6 liters of carbon dioxide are sufficient. After the creation of pneumoperitoneum, the first working trocar is inserted. In fact, this is one of the riskiest stages of the operation, in which the literature reports many of the complications (damage to the main blood vessels, hollow or parenchymal abdominal organs). Each of them will be discussed in detail in the relevant chapter of the guide, so here we will describe only the technique of placing the first trocar. The assistant raises and holds the abdominal wall maximally above the navel with his left hand, the operator holds the abdominal wall below the navel also with the left hand and inserts with the right hand the trocar with a controlled reciprocating rotational movement.

A. Vascular injuries

A 1. Injuries to blood vessels in the abdominal cavity:

Injuries to blood vessels in the abdominal cavity in almost 100% of the cases are associated with the insertion of the first trocar. Most often, the lesions affect the aorta and the right common iliac artery due to their projection immediately below the navel but vessels that may be damaged are the inferior vena cava, the two iliac arteries and veins, and rarely blood vessels of the mesenterium. This serious complication occurs in approximately 0.07-0.4% of all cases./4, 22, 54/ The mechanism of the lesions includes puncture from the Veress needle or the tip of the first trocar, but there are descriptions of incisional injuries at the time of skin incision near the umbilicus. Predisposing factor in the first place are slim patients where the distance from the skin to the front surface of the large blood vessels ranges from 1-1.5 cm. Figure 6 and Figure 7

Figure 6

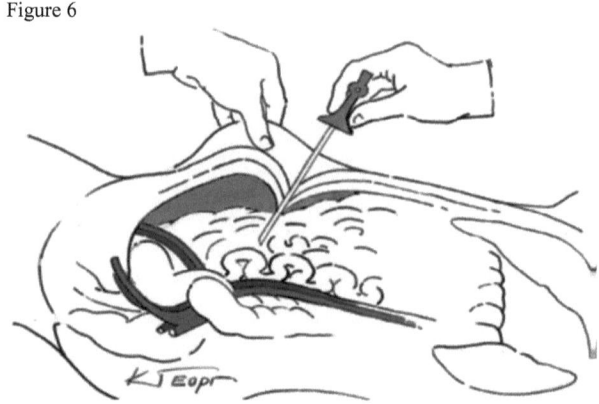

Figure 7

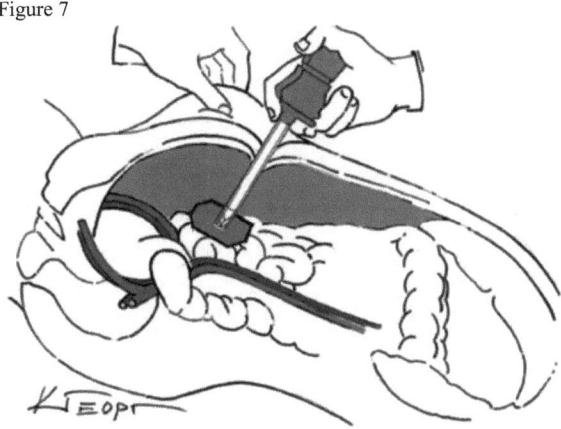

The second predisposing factor is patient with congenital or acquired aortic aneurysms. As a result of such injuries a massive hemorrhage and shock are present. The average rate of mortality in these injuries reaches 28% of the recorded cases. /22, 54, 57/ The clinical manifestation of the complication is dramatic. With the insertion of the laparoscope through the cannula no clear view of the peritoneal cavity is available, and plenty of blood and cloths are visible. In some cases quick "swelling" and "bruising" of the retroperitoneum are observed. Despite intraoperative resuscitation patients present a picture of acute massive haemorrhage, collapse of blood pressure, and increased heart rate. Most appropriate approach is immediate exploratory median laparotomy to specify and control the source of bleeding.

Tips and tricks from senior surgeons:

1. At the beginning of your learning curve with laparoscopic cholecystectomy use opened Hasson technique for placement of the first working trocar.
2. In case you place it using the standard method, strictly follow the instructions:
-   Hold your forearm adjoined to the body to be able to control the pressure force.
-   Make the skin incision larger than the diameter of the trocar. This will allow you to reach the fascia without the use of excessive force.
-   Always use both reciprocating and rotational motion of the wrist at 180 degrees. This provides the best control of the movement of the hand.
3. After placing the laparoscope inspect carefully the mesenterium.

4. In case of diagnosed damage proceed immediately to laparotomy, tamponade and contact a specialist in vascular surgery. In laparotomy leave Veress needle/trocar in place. This way you will most accurately get oriented where the possible damage is.

A 2. Injuries to the blood vessels of the abdominal wall:

The most common cause of hemodynamically significant haemorrhages in/or out of the peritoneal cavity is injury to the lower epigastric artery or vein during insertion of the supplementary (auxiliary) trocars. Usually this complication occurs "subversively" as the inserted cannula presses the ligation and temporarily acts as tamponade to bleeding. At the end of the operation, after removal of the cannula, and moving the patient, it is resumed and can occur in two ways. In the first of them the blood flows into the free peritoneal cavity thus forming a haemoperitoneum. In the second the blood collects in the sheath of the rectus abdominal muscle with the formation of a large hematoma. In either case, this complication may result in huge blood loss, the development of hemorrhagic shock and death of the patient if not detected on time.

The clinical course and manifestation of the complication depend on the time of its registration. Although rare, it can be diagnosed during surgery if the cannula does not "tamponade" effectively the ligation and one can observe continuous flowing at fast drops or trickle of blood in the 5 mm tube in which the grasper is located. This is the most favorable situation for the patient, in which immediate reaction is possible to prevent massive blood loss. In this case, the most correct behavior is to remove the inserted cannula and to extend the incision by 1-2 cm and to make two haemostatic (deep and covering the entire thickness of the abdominal wall) stitches at the top and bottom edges of the original incision under the control of the camera. Figure 8

Figure 8

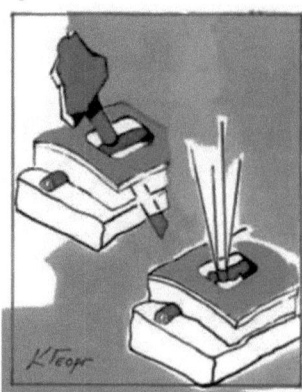

This could be achieved by performing a laparoscopic sutured using Kate straight needle. Figure 9

Figure 9

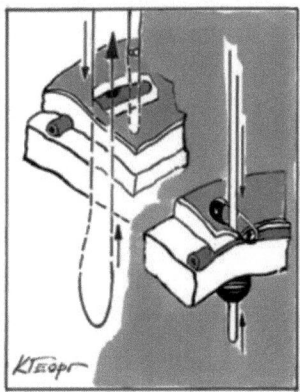

Some authors report a successful control of bleeding by pressing the trocar orifice by the urethral catheter balloon inserted into the cannula./6/ Figure 9

This technique allows temporary hemostasis but does not give us the certainty for complete arrest of bleeding. In the other situations bleeding has a secondary character and the clinical manifestations of hemorrhage are presented by hemorrhage with signs of hemorrhagic shock. The patient has pale skin and mucous membranes, instable hemodynamics, blood pressure is low and the heart rate is increased. In such cases, the condition is often attributed to the "deep general anesthesia" and the effect of drugs, and the right moment to react may be omitted. If the patient has drainage in the bladder bed, it works effectively and the hemorrhage is in the peritoneal cavity, we will obtain accurate and timely information about the complication that has occurred. However, this condition is associated with the mention of the conjunction 'if' several times. In the first place many centers do not routinely place a drain in bladder bed in the absence of indications. In the second place, even when the bleeding is into the peritoneal cavity, the drain can become clogged by a blood clot and drainage is not effective. And thirdly, bleeding may be in the rectus abdominal muscle and there is no formation of haemoperitoneum. That is why the diagnosis of this complication is mainly based on the clinical manifestation and laboratory tests. Changes in blood counts can be monitored in dynamics and are very precise in identifying postoperative bleeding. Any reduction in hemoglobin of more than 10-15 g/l, detected twice (control laboratory error) in the early postoperative period should not carelessly be explained by intraoperative hemodilution by rehydration and the possible source of bleeding should be deliberately sought for. In case of suspicion of such a scenario, a crucial role is played by examination of the abdominal cavity by ultrasound or computer tomography. Both methods are of great informative value with regard to the detection of fluid in the peritoneal cavity or the abdominal wall. After the successful detection of any complication, the most appropriate approach is to carry out emergency relaparoscopy/ laparotomy, final control of the source of bleeding, thorough cleaning of the peritoneal cavity and adequate drainage. Postoperative cares are not different from those of any other patient with postoperative bleeding.

Tips and tricks from senior surgeons:

1. Insert the auxiliary trocars in places remote from the alleged anatomic course of epigastric vessels.

2. Insertion of the trocars must be performed under control of diaphanoscopy using the camera into the abdominal cavity. Close position of the laparoscope of about 1-2 cm from the abdominal wall makes blood vessels clearly distinguishable except in cases of third degree obesity.

3. At least two or three times during the surgery hold your attention of the holes for the trocars while checking for possible bleeding.

4. At the end of the operation, before the removal of the last trocar thoroughly inspect all incisional openings.

5. Always insert 14 Charrière drain into the bladder bed (never harms, and can help a lot).

6. Assign routine blood counts 1-2 hours after surgery. It is not costly and can orient you quickly and accurately what is happening with the patient.

2. Visceral injuries
Injuries to hollow and abdominal parenchymal organs

Damage to the abdominal organs in the creation of pneumoperitoneum has its own characteristics and reaches 0.07-0.7% of common complications in laparoscopic cholecystectomy. /4 , 17, 20, 23/ It usually occurs in patients with prior surgery or inflammation in the peritoneal cavity with postoperative adhesions. This is considerably less frequently observed in patients with normal anatomical relations of the organs in the abdominal cavity.

A. Injuries to hollow abdominal organs

Lesions caused by Veress needle are punctiform and have small diameter, while those caused by the first trocar may have drilling and tearing character, with a larger diameter and the shape of a star. Most characteristic of these injuries is that they remain away from the main field of vision, showing up late with manifestations of incipient or advanced peritonitis. Diagnosis of these iatrogenic injuries at the time of their occurrence is often a consequence of accidental detection of the damaged organ due to limited leakage of contents into the peritoneal cavity. When identified during the actual surgery, there are two approaches to their final remediation. If the expertise and experience of the surgeon allow laparoscopic suture of the injured area, the best option is immediate lesion recovery and completion of cholecystectomy. In case of impossibility for thorough laparoscopic revision of the entire abdominal cavity, as well as lack of experience in laparoscopic suturing technique, the best approach is conversion, restitution of the injured area and completion of cholecystectomy with open abdomen. Unfortunately, in most cases these injuries are noticed on the second or third day of the postoperative period after the intervention, with the manifestations of postoperative peritonitis. Orientation in these cases is very difficult due to the sluggish and gradual course of the peritonitis, the presence of residual gas in the peritoneal cavity from the surgery itself, and the postoperative bowel paresis. The amount of leaked intestinal or other contents is also small, which hinders its identification with the methods of image diagnostics. For these reasons, an exact and timely diagnosis of these iatrogenic lesions is crucial for the successful overcoming of their consequences. Their establishing relies primarily on the clinical judgment of the surgeon and less on objective methods of testing. In these cases what Prof. Lukanov said applies in full measure regarding decisions in emergency surgery - "better act like Don Quixote than like Hamlet". In this sense measures mentioned in the above sections apply as preventive measures for these complications. The specific feature here is the creation of pneumoperitoneum in patients with previous abdominal surgery or suspicion of peritoneal adhesions. One approach is the use of Veress needle, when the initial puncture is made in the left hypochondrium where adhesions are absent. A more popular approach is the use of the open method of Hasson. Most often subjects to injury are small bowel loops, but various departments of the large intestine (colon transversum or colon sigmoideum) as well as the stomach, duodenum, bladder or the uterus in women may be affected/39,40,50,54/.

B. Injuries to parenchymal abdominal organs

Injuries to parenchymal organs during creation of pneumoperitoneum are extremely rare. These are described mainly in cases of hepatosplenomegaly, when part of the liver and spleen are within the range of Veress needle and the trocar. They are manifested by a picture of intra-abdominal hemorrhage, and in case of damage by the trocar blade, hemorrhage can be massive. Diagnosis is easy as the hemorrhage is clearly visible. In liver damage usually control of a bleeding episode is achieved laparoscopically through tamponade of the wounded area and use of local haemostatic agents. Lesions of the spleen are a serious challenge, as an attempt to laparoscopic hemostasis is possible only in small superficial lesions. In cases of deep lacerations of the parenchyma, one should proceed to conversion and splenectomy./40, 54, 67, 68/

Tips and tricks from senior surgeons:

1. In case of suspected peritoneal adhesions and available or established hepatosplenomegaly always use the method of Hasson to create pneumoperitoneum.
2. If during the initial inspection of the peritoneal cavity you detect the presence of adhesions in the vicinity of the first trocar, insert the second working trocar, move the camera in it and thoroughly inspect the peri-umbilical area.
3. During the inspection of the intestinal loops watch out for the appearance of discrete bubbles on the intestinal surface. Often this is the only manifestation of puncture lesion of the intestinal wall.

3. Insufflation of carbon dioxide into the extraperitoneal space. Gas embolism, subcutaneous emphysema, preperitoneal emphysema, pneumomediastinum, pneumothorax.

Insufflation of carbon dioxide into the extraperitoneal space is relatively prevalent condition that does not endanger directly the lives of patients with the exception of cases of gas embolism. Nevertheless it is regarded as a complication requiring appropriate prevention and adequate treatment when present.

A. Gas embolism

An exceptionally rare complication of laparoscopic cholecystectomy, which occurs in direct insufflation of carbon dioxide in a blood vessel with a larger caliber and/or parenchymal organ. The diagnosis is difficult and should be suspected in any patient with abrupt occurence of hypotension, arrhythmia and cardiac arrest. Monitoring of indicators during gas embolism includes higher pressure in the pulmonary artery, increased central venous pressure and increased partial pressure of carbon dioxide in arterial blood. An exact identification of the state is made with transesophageal echocardiography which allows visualization of the gas bubbles in the right heart chambers./19/ Figure 10

Figure 10

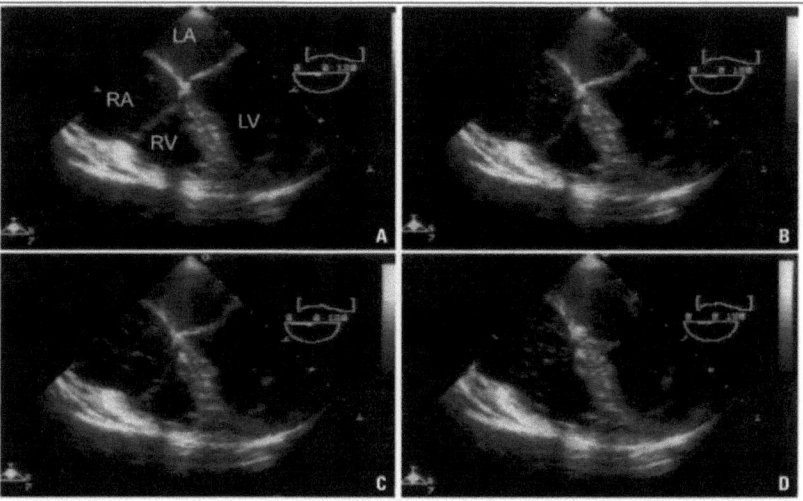

Eun Young Park, Ja-Young Kwon, and Ki Jun Kim, Carbon Dioxide Embolism during Laparoscopic Surgery, Yonsei Med J. 2012 May 1; 53(3): 459–466. /19/

Prevention of the complication is the use of the protocol when inserting Veress needle. Other methods of prevention include - patient in Fauler position with the head tilted back to block access of gas bubbles to cerebral circulation. Maintenance of central venous pressure equal to or higher than the pressure in the peritoneal cavity, and maintaining a positive expiratory end pressure./1, 9, 19/

Therapy of already occurred complication begins with stop of carbon dioxide supply and total peritoneal dessuflation. Ventilation is performed with one hundred percent oxygen. The patient is placed in left lateral Trendelenburg position. A multi-channel central venous catheter is inserted through which the carbon dioxide is aspirated into the right atrium. Some authors quote the positive effect of the application of hyperbaric oxygenation to reduce the amount of gas emboli threefold. In the absence of satisfactory effect of the implemented measures, it is advisable to proceed to emergency thoracotomy, direct cardiac compression and aspiration of carbon dioxide from the cardiac chambers. Unfortunately, mortality remains high in this complication even with a fully adequate treatment and affects 28% of patients./2, 9, 19, 59/

B. Preperitoneal insufflation

The entry of carbon dioxide into the preperitoneal space is predominantly during insertion of Veress needle. Most often the surgeon can be deceived when the needle passes through a thicker subcutaneous layer, which is considered the fascia of the abdominal wall and the click of passing through the actual fascia is thought to be the passage through the parietal peritoneum. In that case the tip of the needle is in the preperitoneal space. In some patients, this space is a looser and lifting of the abdominal wall enables the drop of physiological saline to pass through the needle. Subsequent insufflation with low pressure can also be carried out by actively lifting the abdominal wall, and a uniform tympanic tone can be established in percussion of the abdominal wall. All these factors lead to a rapid increase in pressure to the desired level, apparent ballooning of the abdomen and an impression of successfully formed pneumoperitoneum. Figure 11

Figure 11

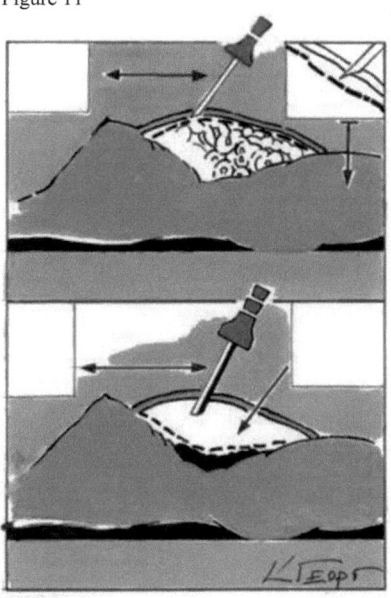

The surgeon becomes aware of the patient status when the laparoscope is inserted. A yellow-orange surface is visible in all directions, with no identification of intraperitoneal organs and structures. There are three approaches to overcome the complication. Aspiration of insufflated gas and insertion of Veress needle at a new location. Insertion of an operative laparoscope with additional working channel through which to bring in scissors to cut the parietal peritoneum. Switching to an open laparotomy./1, 2, 68/ Sometimes carbon dioxide can be insufflated into the omentum maior and the mesenterium. It is presented as "a bulging" omentum with the presence of bubbles on the surface. In certain situations, this may result in interference with the visualization in the peritoneal cavity, but it is not a serious problem if it is not accompanied by a massive haemorrhage.

C. Subcutaneous emphysema

Subcutaneous emphysema is a complication that may manifest itself by a minimum amount of gas around the trocar holes or by massive insufflation of the space from the pelvis minor to the head. In the case of massive subcutaneous emphysema patients resemble the look of the advertising figurine of the tire company "Michelin". The main danger of this complication is due to the abrupt increase in the partial pressure of carbon dioxide, the occurrence of arrhythmia, hypotension, and possible cardiac arrest. Possible reasons for its occurrence in laparoscopic cholecystectomy are several in number. The first is improper positioning of Veress needle in the subcutaneous area. Second is the passing of minimum quantities of gas in retrograde direction around the working trocars. In both cases, generally the amount of carbon dioxide is small and does not pose a clinical problem. In the third case, a large amount of gas can be insufflated into the subcutaneous space during exit of the top of the insufflation cannula out of the peritoneal cavity into the subcutaneous space. This can remain unnoticed by the operating team for a long time because of the cover sheets and the remote position of the insufflation cannula regarding the visual field. Usually the first to signal the complication is the anesthesiologist with information about unusual rise in the partial pressure of carbon dioxide. Examination of the abdominal and chest wall clearly shows the situation in which the patient is. This condition does not require special measures due to the relatively low life-threatening risk for the patient. Of course the position of the insufflation cannula is immediately corrected and ventilation with 100% oxygen is performed. In difficult management of emergent cardiac arrhythmias or respiratory disorders the subcutaneous space may be desufflated using venflon needle of wider diameter. The severely "swollen" subcutaneous layer is punctured in several places and the gas is 'squeezed out'. One should not resort to this measure without reason because of the risk of infection of the subcutaneous tissue. In terms of differential diagnosis one must have in mind possible presence of concomitant pneumomediastinum and/or pneumothorax. Intraoperative radiography is a fast and accurate method to detect the presence of gas in the mediastinum or pleural cavity. If gas is absent in the mediastinum or pleural cavity but is visibly present in the subcutaneous space, the sick are treated as in isolated subcutaneous emphysema.Figure 12

Figure 12 – Massive subcutaneous emphysema without pneumothorax or pneumomediastinum

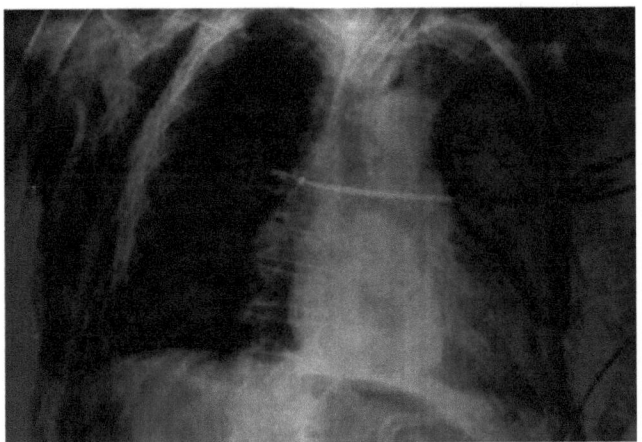

The rapid resorption carbon dioxide leads to definitive overcoming of the complication within 48-72 hours./1, 6/

D. Pneumomediastinum and pneumothorax

We consider these two conditions simultaneously, since in most cases they are observed as a combined complication. At the core of the mechanism of occurrence stands the spread of carbon dioxide through the retroperitoneum or through congenital pores of the diaphragm to the mediastinum or pleural cavity.

Intraoperative diagnosis is difficult because of mechanical ventilation of patients. In some cases one can observe a drop in oxygen saturation, increase in the inspiratory breathing pressure, and attenuated breathig in the involved half of the chest. This complication is usually detected in the early postoperative period after extubation of patients. This is when the lack of breathing in the respective chest half and low oxygen saturation are noticed. Radiography is definitive in the presence of gas in the mediastinum and corresponding pleural cavity. In some cases the pneumomediastinum can precede by minutes and hours the occurrence of pneumothorax. This imposes the need of a control x-ray or CT scan 1-2 hours postoperatively in case of isolated pneumomediastinum to have an exact diagnosis of late or partial pneumothorax. Figure 13 and Figure 14

Figure 13 – Available pneumomediastinum without evidence of pneumothorax

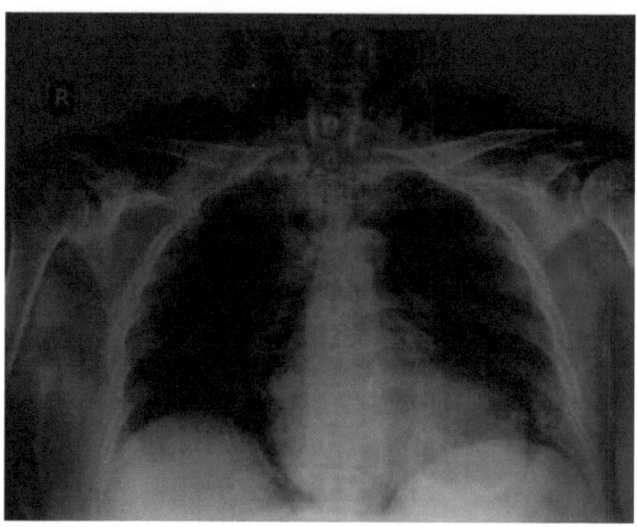

Figure 14 – CT evidence of partial pneumothorax

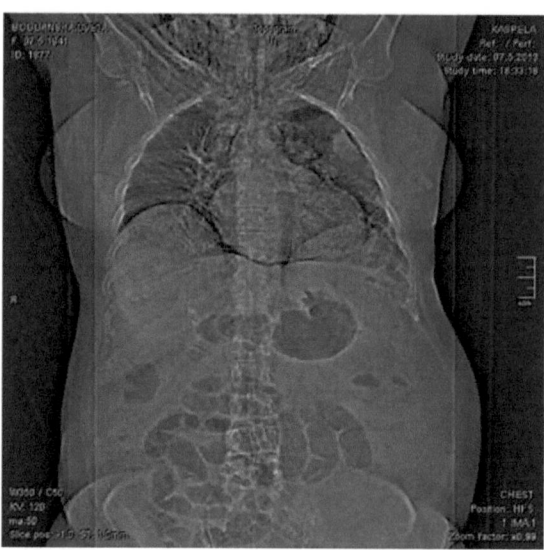

In regard to differential diagnosis the possibility of injury to the trachea in difficult intubation and the emergence of pneumomediastinum and subcutaneous emphysema

in the upper half of the torso should be borne in mind. In such cases, valuable input about the state of the trachea is given performing a tracheoskopy. In the absence of evidence for lesions of the membranous portion of the trachea, the reason should be artifiticial pneumoperiotoneum. Patients with isolated pnevmomediastinum are treated conservatively with antibiotic prophylaxis and active monitoring. In patients with pneumothorax thoracentesis is performed and they are actively aspirated for 48 hours./1, 2, 20, 48/

II. Complications associated with surgical techniques

1. Injuries to hollow abdominal organs

Injuries to hollow viscera related to the specific surgical technique of cholecystectomy are relatively less common than those resulting during the creation of pneumoperitoneum. Most often the site of iatrogenic injury is the duodenum, followed by the stomach and the transverse colon. Predisposing factor for these injuries is the presence of previous or current inflammation of the gall bladder and surrounding tissues. Bladder adhesions with neighboring organs on the one hand make difficult the anatomical dissection of the structures in the triangle of Kalot, on the other hand they change their elasticity from cartilage stiffness to a vulneruble surface. The majority of iatrogenic lesions occur in attempts to "force" detachment of adhesions to the gastric or intestinal wall, as well as excessive use of monopolar coagulation in the same spot.

A. Perforation of the duodenum

Duodenal perforation could be conditionally divided into two main types:
- Duodenal perforation in separating a preceding cholecystoduodenal fistula.
- Duodenal perforation in simple adhesions.

The presence of cholecystoduodenal fistula should be suspected in any case of "rigid" adhesion which may be surrounded on all sides. Figure 15 and Figure 16

Figure 15   Figure 16

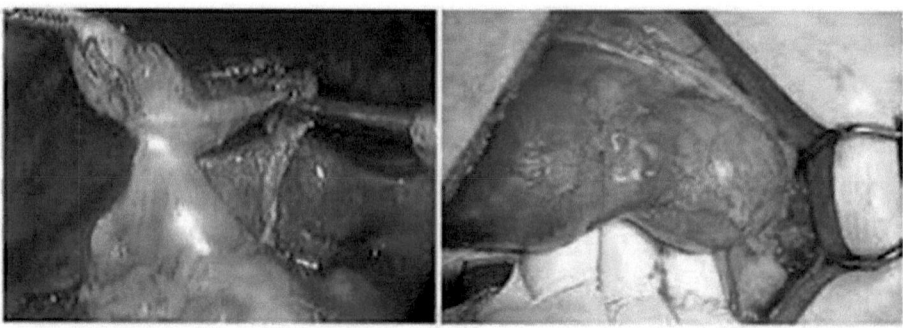

After Sanjeev Kumar Sareen, „Cholecystoduodenal Fistula is not the Contraindication for Laparoscopic Surgery„ World Journal of Laparoscopic Surgery, January-April 2011; 4(1):41-46 /53/

Usually this is a sure sign of the presence of connective tissue tunnel connecting the lumens of the bladder and the duodenum. In those cases it is better to break this bond by means of a stapler, rather than attempting to suture the duodenum after the opening of the fistula. Figure 17 and Figure 18a, Figure 18b, Figure 18c, Figure 18d

Figure 17 –Dividing the fistula with a stapler

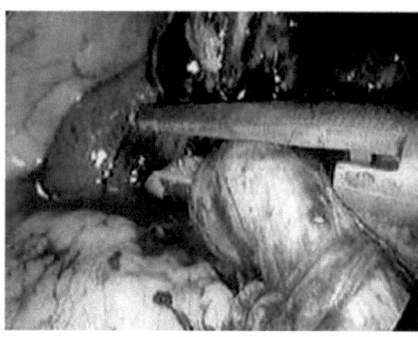

After Sanjeev Kumar Sareen, „Cholecystoduodenal Fistula is not the Contraindication for Laparoscopic Surgery" World Journal of Laparoscopic Surgery, January-April 2011;4(1):41-46 /53/

Figure 18a, Figure 18б, Figure 18c, Figure 18d

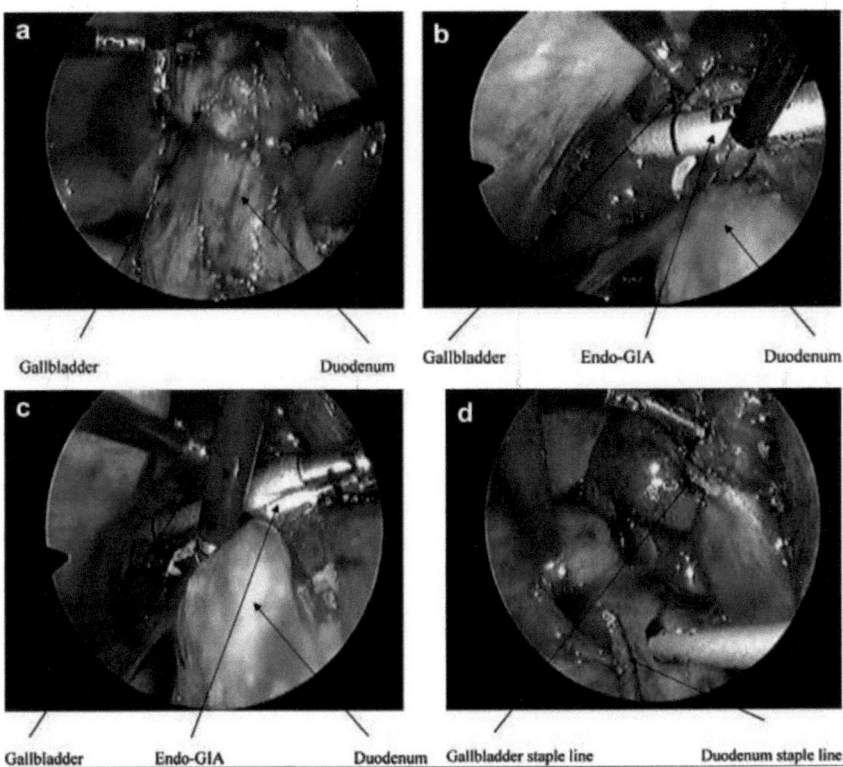

After Leunq E, Kumar P.Bilo-enteric fstula (BEF) at laparoscopic cholecystectomy: Review of ten year's experience.,The Surgeon,Volume 8, Issue 2 , Pages 67-70, April 2010 /32/

In cases of opening the duodenum for dissection of gross adhesions, the integrity of its wall should be restored by laparoscopic or open technique depending on the experience of the team. Unfortunately, in many cases, the lesion may be very small and go unnoticed during surgery. Clinical manifestations occur in the postoperative period with signs of peritonitis or leakage of gastro-duodenal contents through the contact drain if there is one./32, 53/

B. Injury to the colon

The transverse part of the colon is the next target location of iatrogenic lesions due to its frequent involvement as part of the pericholecystic inflammatory process. It is characteristic of these injuries to occur "unexpectedly" for the operator during the release of the bladder from adhesions with the omentum. The colon is deeply "hidden" in these adhesions and their harsh release leads to an opening in the wall of the colon. This damage is usually diagnosed intraoperatively as there is always spill of colonic contents in the operative field. It is recommended to close the lesion with an automatic stapler for the intestinal wall. Laparoscopic suture is also possible with interrupted or continous one layer suture in sufficient experience with laparoscopic suture of tissues, but the method is time-consuming and uncertain. Primary preventive measure regarding damage to the hollow abdominal organs during removal of the gallbladder remains careful dissection of the tissues, exact anatomic orientation, work at a lower grade of the electrocautery system and the provision of clean and clear vision during surgery. Intraoperatively diagnosed injuries should be closed in the first place through laparoscopic stapler and only in extreme cases by tissue sutures. In cases of uncertainty in identifying and/or treating injuries by laparoscopic technique, it is necessary to convert to open surgery, to revise the organs and restore their integrity./1, 6, 23/

Tips and tricks from senior surgeons:

1. When there are adhesions on or around the gallbladder use monopolar coagulation with a power not exceeding 45 watts to dissect them.
2.You can perform successful dissection with the tip of the pump while helping with irrigation and aspiration during the separation of tissues.
3.In case of suspicion of injury to the duodenal wall, insert about 250-300 ml saline colored with methylene blue through a NGT. Even in the smallest lesion, invisible at first glance, you will receive a coloring of the field.
4.If you isolate one part of the stomach, duodenum or colon that are rigidly attached to the gallbladder, do not persevere with dissection to the "end". Whether there is or there is no bile-digestive fistula, the best approach is to divide the adhesion using a laparoscopic stapler.
5.In cases of massive release of adhesions, damage to the serosa layer of parts of the GIT , always end your surgery with drainage of the bladder bed using drain Charrière 24-28 through a 10 mm cannula.

2. Bleeding in the operative field

The main sources of bleeding in the operative field are the liver in the area of gallbladder bed, the cystic artery, the right branch of the proper hepatic artery and very rarely the portal vein or its branches in the area of the triangle of Kalot.

A. Bleeding from the gallbladder bed

This is the most commonly occurring hemorrhage during the operative procedure which is due to its greatest degree to damage of the terminal hepatic arterioles and venules in the underlying parenchyma. Although rare, a source of massive and life-threatening bleeding can also be the large branches of the middle hepatic vein when passing at 0.5 -1 cm depth in the bed of the gallbladder. The mechanism of damage to these blood vessels is either mechanical or due to heat injury during dissection of the gallbladder from the liver parenchyma in the region of the fifth segment. In the ideal cases, this dissection is performed in subserose plan with no bleeding. Unfortunately, quite often this maneuver is difficult on the one hand because of "intact" bladder with extremely thin wall, and the other- because of concomitant destructive inflammation with loss of the subserous plan. Another predisposing factor is the presence of accompanying liver cirrhosis with portal hypertension. The nature of the bleeding in these cases is from mild with the appearance of dew-like drops of dark blood to massive in which dark-colored blood flows like a "gutter" and fills in quicklyl the sub-hepatic space./16, 27, 31, 41, 43, 56, 62/ Diagnosis of the source of bleeding is relatively easy because it is located in the center of the visual field. There are various methods for temporary and definitive hemostasis of bleeding from the bladder bed, which depend on the degree of bleeding. In the mild forms most often hemostasis occurs spontaneously and does not require control by surgical methods. In other cases, the following methods of hemostasis may be used:

Monopolar electrocoagulation with the back of the disector or a specific instrument ("elephant step") until bleeding is stopped. In case of failure bipolar coagulation with laparoscopic bipolar forceps can be applied. In almost 90% of cases it is sufficient to achieve total hemostasis. In persistent bleeding the source of bleeding can also be clamped with the tool tip, the aspiration probe, a grasper with entrapped "beans", or by placing radiopaque gauze tape for a period of 2-3 minutes in the peritoneal cavity. In addition to the above method various sealants, sponges and nets containing thrombin can be used with excellent results. It is important to note that attempts to laparoscopic suture or clipping in the bladder bed are doomed to failure and can only delay the necessary measures and lead to hemodynamically significant blood loss. In case all of the above methods fail to control the bleeding, one should proceed to conversion, identification of the source of bleeding and its eradication.

B. Bleeding from the cystic artery

This is less common due to the special attention given to identifying, clipping and cutting of the artery or its branches as a key step in laparoscopic cholecystectomy. However, there are many cases of conversion indicated by hemorrhage with a source the cystic artery, which cannot be controlled laparoscopically. The causes of this complication are:

1. Numerous variations in the separation and the course of the cystic artery to its entry into the gallbladder. Figure 19 presents the main variations.

Figure 19 – Variations in the course and separation of the cystic artery

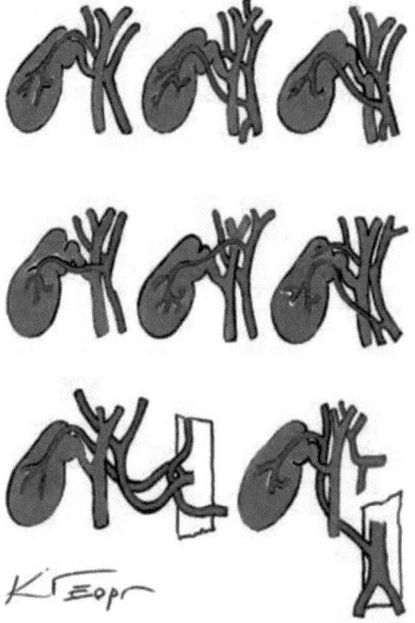

2. Divergence of normal anatomic relationships of the structures in the triangle of Kalot due to available acute or chronic inflammation of the gallbladder, malignant degeneration of the gallbladder.

3. Difficult dissection of the structures in the triangle of Kalot due to hepatomegaly, cirrhosis of the liver, adhesions from previous surgery.

4. "Short" course of the artery from the separation from ramus dexter to the gallbladder - 0.5 to 1 cm.

Causes of complication can be divided into the following groups:

1. Injury to the trunk or branches of the cystic artery during dissection before positioning of the clips.
2. Incorrect positioning of clips with leaving some of the arterial trunk free.
3. Slippage of a clip positioned during the time of surgery.
4. Rupture of a "short" artery in rough bladder lift.

Depending on the flow bleeding may range from slightly "trickling" to massive with violating the visualization of the operative field. It should be borne in mind that in the destructive forms of acute cholecystitis, especially in gangrene of the gallbladder, there is concomitant partial or total arterial thrombosis. Absence of bleeding upon discontinuation of the trunk in these cases does not free the surgeon from the obligation to perform clipping or ligation to prevent the occurrence of secondary hemorrhage. Often the initiation of the cystic artery lesion is represented by a sudden loss of cleanliness of field due to soiling of the tip of the laparoscope located in the immediate vicinity of the site of operation. In such a case it is particularly important to gain self control, to clean the laparoscope, to preserve the position of the assistant, and to start secondary inspection of the field long in advance before the insertion of laparoscope in the peritoneal cavity. In the majority of cases the source of bleeding is clearly visible and can be carefully and selectively controlled. When the bleeding flow rate is lower the identification of the complication is relatively easy and it can be controlled by various methods. Of particular importance is the need for precision and selectivity in the control of bleeding due to the risk of damage to other structures in the gross and massive grip and clipping of the source of bleeding. /6, 28, 57/ For clarity in choice of decision behavior in different flow rate bleeds from the cystic artery the scheme in Figure 20 can be used.

Figure 20 – Schematic behavior in different flow rate bleeding from the cystic artery

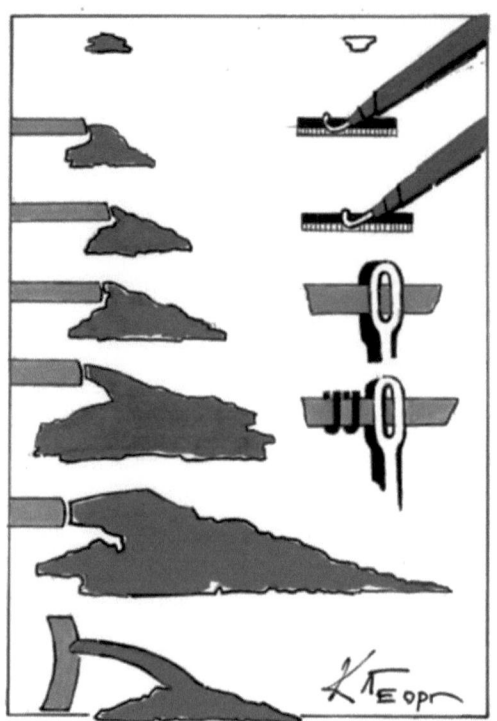

C. Injuries to the right branch of the proper hepatic artery

Lesions of the right branch of the proper hepatic artery as a rule occur in cases where it passes near the infundibulum of the bladder and the course of the cystic artery itself is "short". In almost all cases, the right branch is perceived as the cystic artery and is clopped and cut. In cases of partial lesion of the wall bleeding is massive with high capacity and requires immediate conversion. When clipped and cut, severe ischemia of the right hepatic lobe occurs with postoperative disturbance of liver function. Sometimes this can result in necrosis of the right lobe and subsequent abscesses. This requires the cystic artery dissection to be made in close proximity to the wall of the gallbladder. /1, 6, 17/

D. Injuries to the portal vein or its branches

Injuries to the portal vein or its branches is casuistry. Several isolated cases have been described, which as a rule are accompanied by massive life-threatening hemorrhages and are subject to control only after immediate conversion. Of the other part the literature presents numerous reports of bleeding from extremely dilated bladder venous vessels and plexuses in cases of portal hypertension due to liver cirrhosis. The wall of venous vessels is extremely thin and "fragile". Bladder veins which in ordinary cases are not visible or coagulate, in these patients have a diameter up to 0.5 cm, they are tense and rupture easily even in the most careful attempts to dissect them. Bleeding is massive, quickly becomes hemodynamically significant, and requires immediate conversion and final control. In this aspect, we consider necessary to refine the indications for laparoscopic cholecystectomy in such patients. It remains an option for cases of emergency indications and extreme caution is required when working in the triangle of Kalot. The principle of instrumental readiness for laparotomy should not be underestimated. /16, 20, 23, 27/

Tips and tricks from senior surgeons:

1.In bleeding from the bed of the gallbladder, which is not controlled by mono or bipolar coagulation, insert into the peritoneal cavity gauze tape with radiopaque thread and firmly press the bleeding area for 2-3 min.

2.After separation and clipping of the cystic artery, and when starting the subserous separation, watch out carefully for other vascular structure. If you are working high near the gallbladder, the severed vessel could be only one of the branches of the artery. There is the possibility that there is a second one behind it. This is the most common cause of bleeding during the procedure.

3.If the bleeding in the hilus is massive "grab" it with atraumatic grasper, and hold it in this position until the rapid transition to conversion.

3. Injuries to the extrahepatic bile ducts

Iatrogenic lesions of the extrahepatic bile ducts during laparoscopic cholecystectomy appears to be the "Achilles heel" of this procedure. This is the complication that although by a small percentage exceeds the same complication in open surgery. For a long time it was the main factor obstructing the expansion of indications for performance of laparoscopic cholecystectomy. At this stage, it remains one of the most severe and life-threatening conditions that accompany this methodology. /13, 14, 17/

Predisposing factors for its occurrence are:
1. Anatomical variations in the course and branches of the extrahepatic bile ducts – Figure 21

Figure 21 - Anatomical variations of the biliary tract

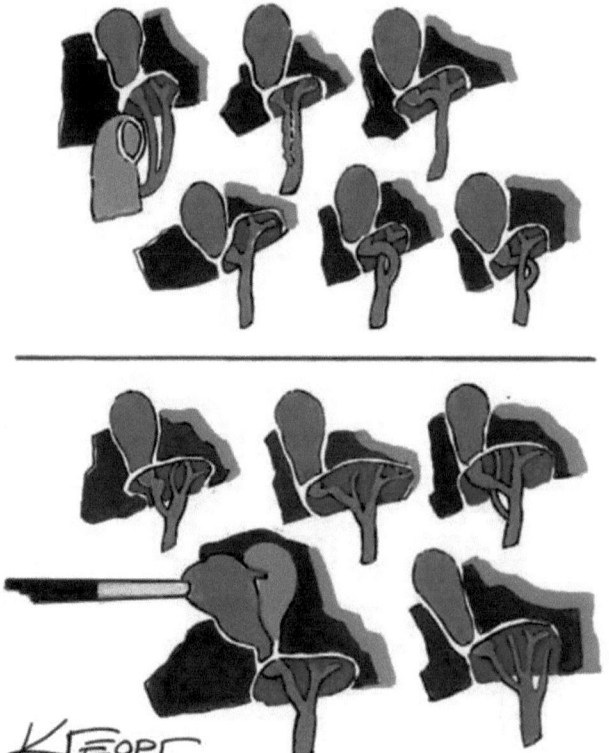

2. Violated anatomical relationships in the triangle of Kalot from acute and/or chronic inflammation of the gallbladder and the surrounding tissues. Presence of fibrosis and adhesions in the hilus from previous surgical interventions. Presence of comorbidities with marked hepatomegaly.

3.Insufficient experience of the surgeon - in the performance of less than 20 surgeries per year the rate of iatrogenic lesions is significantly higher compared to that of surgeons with more experience.

4.Impaired perception of the two-dimensional image that prevents adequate assessment of the situation in depth.

5.The presence of bleeding during the "rough" intervention and attempts control it nonselectively are the most common prerequisites for combined lesions of blood and bile vessels in laparoscopic cholecystectomy.

Direct reasons for injuries to extrahepatic tract most often are mechanical cutting (full or partial) in perceiving them as bladder ducts, a mechanical narrowing (full or partial) by the use of clips, a combination of the two mechanisms, thermal injury while working with electrosurgical tools on or near the bile ducts. The two most common mechanism of mechanical cutting or clipping of the common bile duct are associated with misinterpretation of the anatomy of the structures in the triangle of Kalot, due to inadequate traction and exposure of the gallbladder./7, 13, 14, 21, 25/ Figure 22 a, b, c and 23 a, b show the mechanisms of iatrogenic injuries.

Figure 22 a, b, c

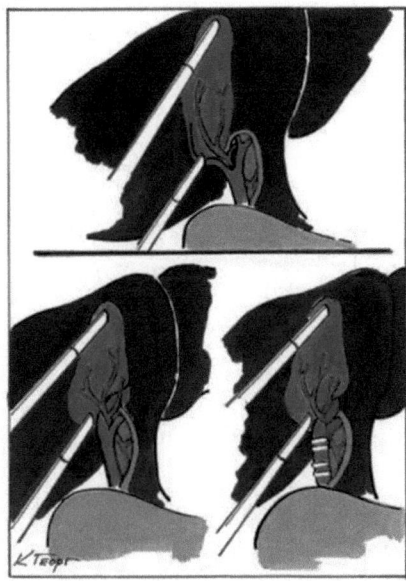

a - The best method for bladder traction and exposure of structures in the triangle of Kalot. Besides in upward direction, traction should be performed in lateral direction as well.

b - Traction is shown only in the upward direction, in which the common bile duct is perceived as long ductus cysticus.

c - The mechanism of clipping of the common bile duct is shown, which is perceived as ductus cysticus.

Figure 23 a, b

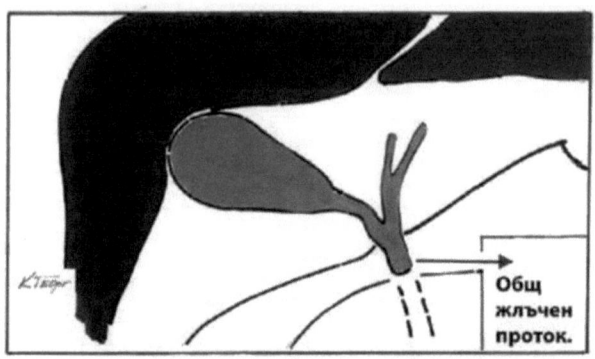

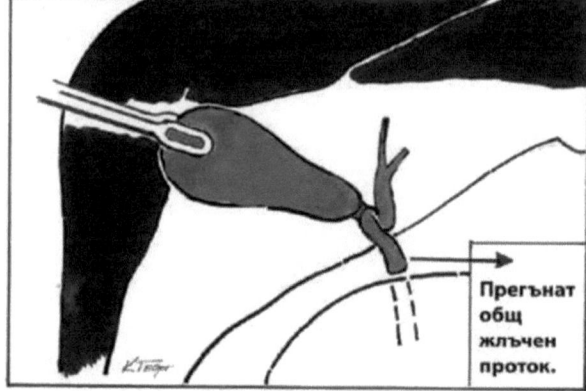

Text in the picture above – common bile duct. Text in the picture below – Kinked common bile duct.

a - The portion of the common bile duct is shown, which can be "pulled out" in massive traction

b - The pulled out area is seen, which is subject to clipping and cutting.

The type and extent of early or late lesions of the bile ducts has been summarized in many different classifications. At present the most common and widely accepted is Bismuth's classification, modified by Strasberg, which is targeted at the possibility for correction of lesions./58/ Figure 24

Figure 24

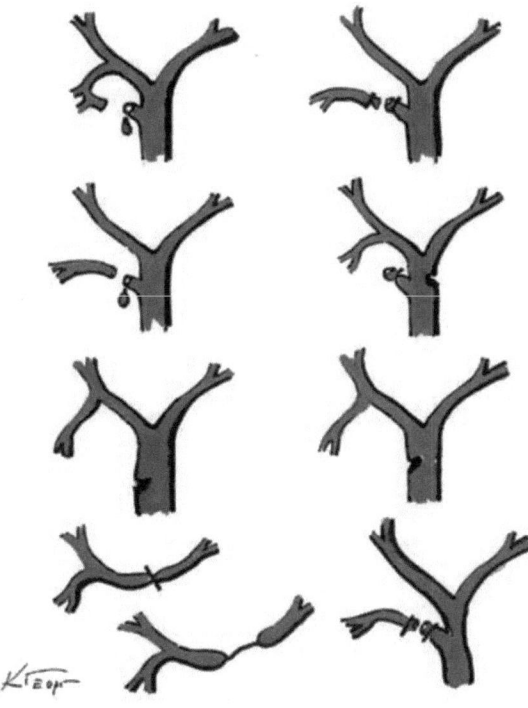

Type A – Leakage of bile from a small bile duct connected to ductus hepaticus communis. For example, leakage from the stump of ductus cysticus, accessory bile duct, etc.

Type B – Occlusion of an aberrant bile duct.

Type C – Leakage of bile from an aberrant duct unrelated to ductus hepaticus communis.

Type D – Lateral lesion of the common bile duct.

Type E – Circumferent lesion of the common bile duct from Class I to Class V after Bismuth.

Diagnosis of these lesions is intraoperative in the smaller number of cases, and postoperative for most of them.

A. Intraoperative identification of extrahepatic biliary duct injuries is difficult because of operator error on the "rightness" of his current actions on the one hand, and on the other hand - because of the low flow rate of bile leakage in the presence of open ducts. In the majority of cases of such lesions found during surgery, it is based on two important circumstances. In the first case the operator and the assistants encounter an "unusual" anatomical findings such as the presence of two lumens of the cut "cystic" duct (cutting of the common hepatic and cystic ducts), presence of "accessory" cystic duct which appears in the ongoing dissection of the bladder (cut common hepatic or bile duct and reaching one of the two hepatic ducts. In the second case, the reason for the identification becomes the establishment of bile leakage in the operative field./21, 25, 26/ Analysis of the situation results in adequate correction of the complication. First step is to procede to conversion and thorough investigating of the biliary tree. Valuable help in this respect is intraoperative cholangiography. The purpose of the immediate correction consists of three main items.

1. Restoration of the integrity and continuity of the biliary tract
2. Termination of any bile leak.
3. Performing of tension-free anastomosis.

In cases of injury to a bile duct with a diameter of less than 3 mm which drains only one segment on intraoperative cholangiography, simple ligation may be performed without risk of biliary obstruction.

Duct with a diameter of more than 3 mm is generally drain more than one segment, and in case of cutting require implantation into the biliary tree. In lesion of the common hepatic or bile duct our behavior depends on the extent of the injury and its distance from the bifurcation. Upon injury of less than 50% of the diameter of non-thermal genesis, the lesion can be restored by an interrupted suture with single resorbable monofilament steach № 0000. Restoration is obligatory accompanied by the insertion of a relieving Kerr drainage through a hole different from that of iatrogenic lesion. In case of injury to more than 50% of the circumference or total interruption, the continuity of the biliary drainage must be restored by bilio-enteric anastomosis.

In case of injury of the distal end of the common bile duct, there are two alternatives.

1. Performing a terminolateral choledoho-duodenostomy. Once ligation of the distal end of the common bile duct is made, one should proceed with one layer termino-lateral anastomosis with interrupted or continuous suture with absorbable

monofilament steachesa № 0000. As the anastomosis has to be tension free, mobilization of the duodenum after Kocher is obligatory. The main disadvantage of this technique is that it can not be completely free of tension. In case of any insufficiency we face the difficult situation of mixed biliary and duodenal fistula. For this reason it has been abandoned by almost all authors and exists more as a theoretical option.

2. The second alternative is to carry out terminolateral choledohojejunostomy a modo Roux. A major feature of this technique is the maintenance of an adequate blood supply to the proximal end of ductus choledochus. For this purpose, it is advisable to avoid the massive longitudinal dissection as it terminates its nutrition. This anastomosis is completely free of tension and shows much better results both in the short and long term.

In case of injury to the common hepatic duct there is only one option – hepatico-jejunostomy a modo Roux. In both of the above scenarios it is good to be aware of the positive effect of placing a protecting stent.

Tips and tricks from senior surgeons:

1.In the intraoperative diagnosis of damage to the bile ducts, first assign completion of surgery to another colleague. The tension of the procedure itself and frustration of iatrogenicity affect the proper behavior in terms of future actions.

2.In the absence of a surgeon with experience in hepatobiliary surgery stop the biliary hemorrhage into the peritoneal cavity, drain the bile ducts outside it and refer the patient to a third level hepatobiliary center. For best results especially in the long term the experience of the surgeon performing the reconstruction is a crucial factor.

3. In deciding to perform the reconstruction of the site, use a termino- lateral mucomucous hepatico-jejunostomy a modo Roux. It is wide enough, and the wall of the ductus hepaticus is better vascularised. Protect the anastomosis with a stent.

B. Diagnosis of lesions in the postoperative period

The majority of cases of iatrogenic injury of the biliary tract are diagnosed during the postoperative period./21, 25, 26, 29/ These are presented mainly by two types of clinical manifestation:

1.Occurrence of obstructive jaundice.

As an independent manifestation of obstructive jaundice in the early postoperative period is due to the obstruction of the bile duct because of ligation or clipping. In the late postoperative period (more than four weeks to six months), it is the consequence of the development of strictures.

2.Occurrence of bilioperitoneum manifested by diffuse biliary peritonitis or localised biloma. In the case of drainage into the operative field, leaks of bile are identified in varying amounts in the drain itself or around it through the incisional opening. Iatrogenic injury to the bile duct should be suspected in any patient with problematic and atypical course of the postoperative period. Ignoring signs such as persistent pain in the upper part of the abdomen 3-4 days postoperatively, available fever, elevated transaminases, alkaline phosphatase, total and/or direct bilirubin result in delayed diagnosis and less options for adequate behavior. In case of suspicion of such complication, it is necessary to clarify the state of the peritoneal cavity (diffuse or limited available peritonitis, presence of non-infected biloma), and the condition of the biliary tract. The use of abdominal ultrasound, CT, MRI, ERCP or PTC gives us sufficient and reliable information on the complication. After the diagnosis of iatrogenic lesion of the biliary tract, the behavior strategy follows three main objectives:

1. Eradication and control of existing infection in the peritoneal cavity. The inflammatory process except its general pathogenic effect is a prerequisite for the formation of fibrosis in the liver hilus, which enormously hinders correction actions regarding lesions of the biliary tract. Administration of broad-spectrum antibiotics and drainage of the available biliary collections in the peritoneal cavity (percutaneous or by laparotomy) lead to the realization of the first objective. Once this is achieved the need for other emergency interventions is eliminated. There is categorical evidence that attempts for surgery on the biliary tract in the early period after the establishment of iatrogenicity have significantly worse outcomes than the deferred and properly planned ones. This behaviour is guided by the poor general condition of the patient and the pronounced swelling of the tissues in the liver hilus.

2. The second objective is clear and precise imaging of the biliary tract by cholangiography. This can be done through ERCP or PTC. In such cases, preference is given to PTC due to the possibility of a more detailed and accurate representation of the intrahepatic bile ducts and the state of the bifurcation. Moreover, percutaneous drainage provides pressure drop in the biliary tree, acts as a permanent biliary drainage and can be used for biliary reconstruction as perioperative drainage. In some cases of partial lesions of the biliary tree with preserved continuity, ERCP with stenting or PTC are sufficient for the final remediation of the lesion.

3. The third objective is the establishment of sustainable and effective biliary-enteric anastomosis. If the lesion is less than 2 cm away from the bifurcation or involves it, we recommend the performance of hepatico-jejunostomy a modo Roux with mucomucous manner and long-term stenting of both hepatic ducts. If the lesion is more than 2 cm from the bifurcation in the distal direction, the same protection of the same anastomosis can be used with Kerr drainage and without stenting of the hepatic ducts. High proximal lesions with available tissue deficiency of bile ducts present a particular challenge. Some authors describe excellent results in segmentectomy of IV and V segments for disclosure of sufficient length of hepatic ducts and especially of the left one which is suitable for anastomosis. A preliminary condition is assessment of the biliary drainage of the passageways of the right lobe to the left hepatic duct by preoperative cholangiography. The experience of the team has a major role in the good short and long-term results in the performance of these reconstructions.Therefore, it is highly recommended to surgeons without such qualifications after diagnosis of such iatrogenic lesions to complete the first objective of the immediate tasks for overcoming the emergency status of the patients, and after that to refer them to specialized hepatobiliary centers for final treatment./30, 33, 42, 44, 46, 60, 63, 64, 69/

Tips and tricks from senior surgeons:

1.Provide external biliary drainage and sanitation of the perineal cavity of the patient.

2.Refer him for further evaluation and rereconstruction to an established center in hepatobiliary surgery to achieve good long-term results.

3.If you are determined to restore the biliary-enteric drainage, strictly follow these rules:

A.   Dissect the proximal end of the bile duct (ducts) with extreme tenderness and delicacy at not more than 5 mm in order to maintain their adequate blood supply.

B.   If you are close to or at the bifurcation itself, use the termino- lateral anastomosis, protected by drainage a modo Witzel. For an incomplete lesion in the middle third, restore the integrity of the duct, by protecting the suture with plastic prosthesis 10 Charrière which has to be removed endoscopically after 30 days.

C.   Use trans-mesocolic access to the jejunal loop as jejuno-jejunostomy has to be done at about 30 cm and length of 50-60 cm from the ligament of Treitz. This will provide a free drainage of pancreatic juices and will prevent them from mixing with bile near the biliary-digestive anastomosis.

D.   Protect the biliary digestive anastomosis by stents or Kerr drainage depending on its location.

C.   Prevention of iatrogenic lesions of the biliary tree

Methods for prevention (prophylaxis) of iatrogenic damage of bile passageways are discussed in depth since the advent of laparoscopic surgery and have undergone a number of corrections in an attempt to find an adequate algorithm. The discussion continues at present apriori these damages are considered to be avoidable, but in an anonymous survey surgeons report that more than 70% of them are unavoidable./37/ The main factor leading to iatrogenicity of bile ducts is misidentification of the structures of the biliary tree. In this context, emphasis is placed on methods to prevent this erroneous anatomical identification. The only structures to be clipped and cut during laparoscopic cholecystectomy are ductus cysticus and the cystic artery. Various methods have been described aimed at their secure identification. These methods are based on three surgical techniques - infundibular technique, the critical view of safety technique and intraoperative cholangiography.

C.1. The infundibular technique

The infundibular technique represents dissection of the infundibular segment of the gallbladder to its presentation in the form of a funnel connecting distally with ductus cysticus. The dissection is carried out from the infundibilum downwards to ductus cysticus or in reverse order. It is based on receiving a three-dimensional image of the "funnel" resulting from the passage of the ductus cysticus in the infundibulum of the gallbladder./37/ The disadvantage of this technique lies in the frequent situation in which the common bile duct often passes closely to the infundibulum of the gallbladder in cases of inflammation and short hidden ductus cysticus. The situation results in the so called "false picture of the funnel". Figure 25 a, b

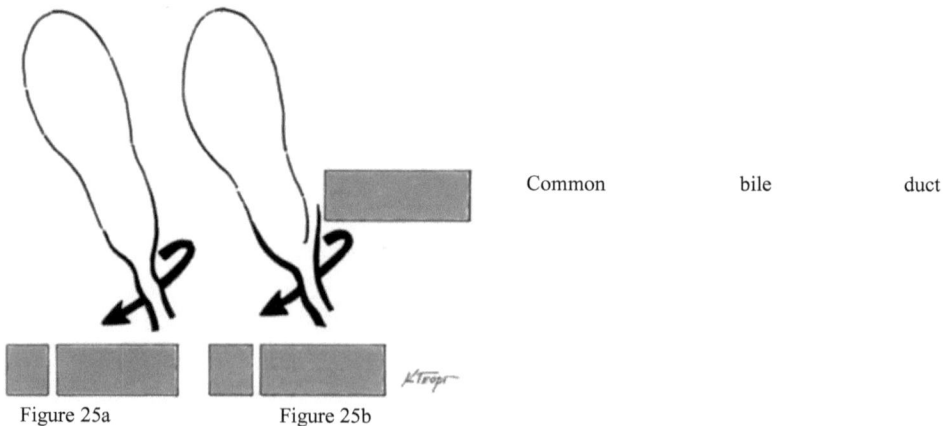

Common   bile   duct

Figure 25a   Figure 25b

This visual deception occurs in the presence of acute destructive inflammatory process, a large concrement in the pocket of Hartman, adhesions between the common bile duct and the gallbladder infundibulum. The result of misinterpretation usually is cutting of the common bile duct.

C.2. Critical view of safety

Critical View of Safety (CVS) - the technique, described by Strasberg, is based on a thorough dissection in the triangle of Kalot to receive two pure structures passing into the gallbladder - the cystic duct and the cystic artery. /58/ The dissection is followed by the release of the lower half of the gallbladder from the liver bed. At this point we can inspect from all sides the "merging" of the two identified structures in the gallbladder. Figure 26 a,b

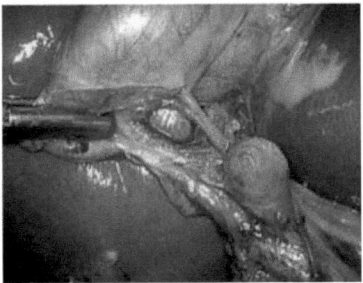

Figure 26a

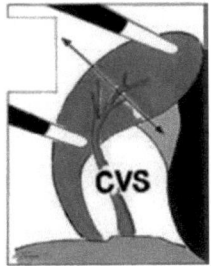

Figure 26b

The identification of the common bile ductIt is considered unnecessary. Failure to obtain clear presentation of the two structures and the inability to inspect them from all sides is considered by Strasberg for an absolute indication for conversion.Since the introduction of this technique many authors shared their results from using it successfully./37, 58, 62, 65, 66/

C.3. The third preventive measure is the use of routine intraoperative cholangiography

Its purpose is to depict the biliary tree as an entity. Figure 27

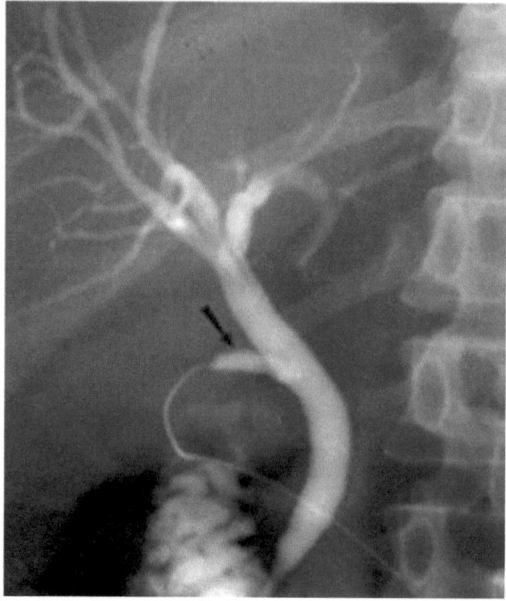

Figure 27 – Normal cholangiography

A number of articles have been devoted to the benefits of this preventive measure, and most of the authors emphasize the target of halving the incidence of damage to the bile duct./37, 38, 39, 62, 66/ The main disadvantage of this method is the need for specific knowledge for the correct interpretation of cholangiography. Misperceptions of the common bile duct as the ductus cysticus and its incision to insert the cholangiographic catheter is an iatrogenic lesion by itself. Figure 28

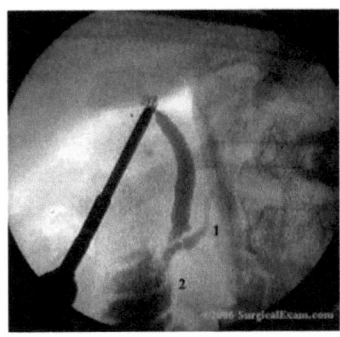

Figure 28

It shows a cholangiography in which the common bile duct is wrongly recognized as ductus cysticus. It has been clipped in the proximal part, an incision is made on the front wall and cholangiography is carried out. A typical picture of a full display of the distal ductus choledochus can be seen and passage of contrast agent into the duodenum without display of the proximal part of common bile and common hepatic duct and the intrahepatic bile ducts. In cases of misinterpretation of the cholangiography image iatrogenic lesions of the common bile duct are not uncommon. Nevertheless in all published series of studies a reduction in cases of damaged bile ducts by a half is reported in the routine use of intraoperative cholangiography. It remains a valuable tool in the so-called "difficult" cases. /37, 38, 39, 62, 66/

In the last year various other techniques for correct anatomical identification of the structures in the triangle of Kalot were reported. Some of them are based on the use of fluorescent stains that are extremely expensive, while others are based on the use of popular colorants such as methylene blue. In these the gallbladder is initially perforated by a Veress needle, then bile is aspirated and the corresponding colorant is administered into the bladder. These techniques are still new and there is no statistically significant and reliable literature data on the benefits of their use./37, 66/

There are also publications describing the method of "subtotal cholecystectomy" as a way out of a situation in which the differentiation of anatomical structures is impossible to achieve. These authors argue that the conversion in these cases does not result in better orientation than the laparoscopic one. There are reports on several dozens of patients with good long-term results./37/

The human factor and iatrogenic damage of the biliary tree.

It is based on on the "human factor" approach described by Reason in highly responsible activities such as the organization of air traffic and the nuclear industry./37/ According to this approach, the surgeon with the lowest risk of iatrogenicity is described as a person aware of unpleasant surprises, adopting colleague advice, ready to change his original hypothesis, knowing the signs and effects of fatigue, time pressure and the anxiety of "presenting his surgical technique". According to Hunter, the team approach is a good preventive measure, as it suggests not to clip and cut cystic duct until each team member is sure of its correct identification./37/

4. Injuries to the diaphragm and the pleura.

Injuries to the diaphragmatic dome and the parietal pleura are very rare complications that occur only in the right side and depend on two main etiologic factors. The first case of injury of the diaphragm and pleura is purely mechanical and occurs during extreme pulling and lifting of the gallbladder over the liver. "Slipping out" of the bladder from the clamping grasper leads to sudden unintended movement of the tool in the direction of the diaphragm, when the muscle part and adjacent pleura are pierced. In the second case the mechanism of the lesion is mixed - mechanical and thermal. It is most commonly obtained by dissection of the gallbladder from the liver bed by a dissecting "hook" by monopolar coagulation and cutting. The assistant holds up the gallbladder until it approaches closely the diaphragm. Upon dissection with the "hook" and the activated electrocautry, careless and uncontrollable movement of the tool results in contact with the diaphragm and its instantaneous puncture together with the pleura from the electrocoagulation. Besides the immediate occurrence of pneumothorax, the literature describes a case with the massive hemopneumotorax based on ruptured adhesions between the parietal pleura and the diaphragmatic surface./1, 5, 48/ Figure 29a,b

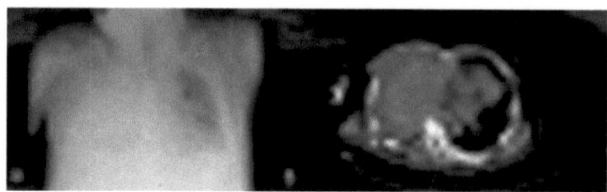

Figure 29a   Figure 29b

Predisposing factors for these injuries are "technically" difficult cholecystectomies against a destructive acute inflammation of the gallbladder or old chronic sclerosing inflammation converting the gallbladder into a "stone". Major predisposing factor of course is the experience of the surgeon and the team. Diagnosis of this lesion is impossible intraoperatively due to the artificial ventilation of patients during surgery. It can only be suspected during such an episode during the surgery. After extubation of the patient chest x-ray is performed still on the operating table with a the mobile apparatus. In the presence of pneumothorax or hemopneumotorax, aspiration drainage of the pleural cavity is immediately necessary. Treatment outcomes are generally excellent if rules for the postoperative period are followed.

Tips and triks from senior surgeon:

1. Perform traction of the gallbladder except in direction above the liver and laterally, also "outwards" from the abdominal wall. This will prevent the sudden drop out of the bladder and rupture of the diaphragm.
2. In the final dissection of the gallbladder from the liver bed, move the grasper from the infundibulum and attach the gallbladder to its fundus. Pull up and towards the abdominal wall so that you move it away from the diaphragm.
3. In case of contact of a tool with activated coagulation with the diaphragmatic surface, always assign chest x-ray after extubation. This can help you to diagnose a clinically undetectable pneumothorax.

5. Obstruction of the bile duct by residual gallstones.

Symptoms of obstructive jaundice occurring as a result of residual gallstones after laparoscopic cholecystectomy may occur in the first few postoperative days up to to 2 years after the operation. Residual gallstones according to literature are concretion that have passed from the gallbladder into the common bile duct before or during surgery./20, 23, 29/ As a general rule, patients with residual gallstones do not have any history, laboratory or examination preoperative data for available choledocholithiasis. Figure 30

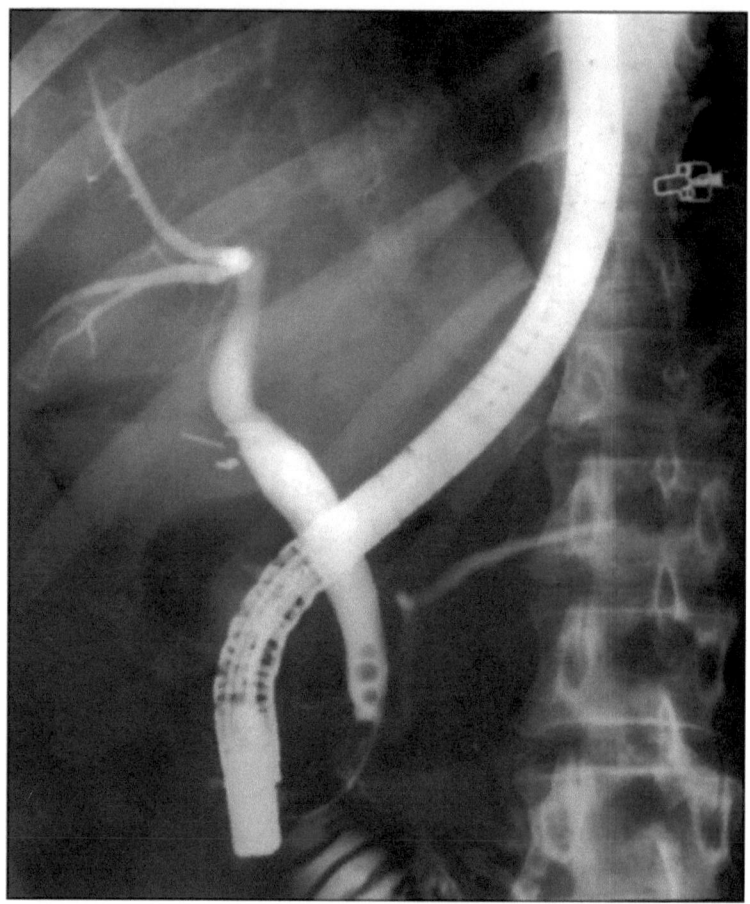

Figure 30 - Residual gallstones

Predisposing factors for this complication include: presence of multiple gallbladder calculi sized 2-3 mm., short and wide ductus cysticus, harsh handling on the gallbladder. Calculi can be found in the common bile duct before surgery (silent stones) but can pass into it during surgery. Usually gallstones that were in the common bile duct before laparoscopic cholecystectomy have theirclinical manifestation later, which is provoked by other factors: dietary error, virus infection. While gallstones passed during cholecystectomy may manifest clinically immediately after the procedure. Obstruction of the common bile duct results in the onset of jaundice on the second postoperative day, and complete obstruction may be manifested with symptoms of biliary peritonitis in leakage of bile through the cystic duct stump regardless of the clipping. Diagnosis of residual gallstones is best done by

ERCP. Besides being a diagnostic method endoscopic cholangiopancreatography plays the role of a therapeutic method. "Broad" sphincterotomy and extraction of gallstones represent the gold standard for treatment of this common complication. /62, 67, 68/ In case of impossibility to refer patients to an ERCP center for various reasons, an alternative is to perform a laparotomy, bile duct exploration, extraction of gallstones and completion of the surgery with Kerr drainage or choledocho-duodeno-anastomosis. Prevention of problems associated with the presence of residual gallstones is based on the performance of routine intraoperative cholangiography. /38/

We have registered 18 cases of unsuspected gallstones in the common bile duct during routine cholangiography in our center for the last two years. This allows extraction of the calculi to be carried out intraoperatively by a balloon catheter, or choledohoscopy. Figure 31

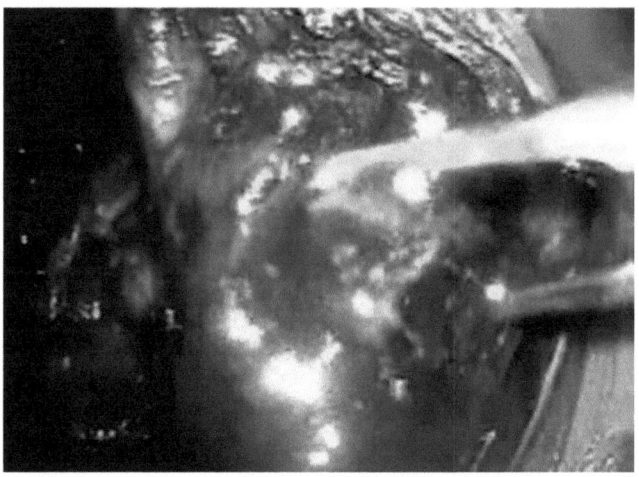

Figure 31 – Extraction of concrements from the common bile duct

In all 18 patients we achieved complete cleansing of gallstones and completion of cholecystectomy laparoscopically by primary suture of common bile duct incision - ideal choledochotomy. Figure 32

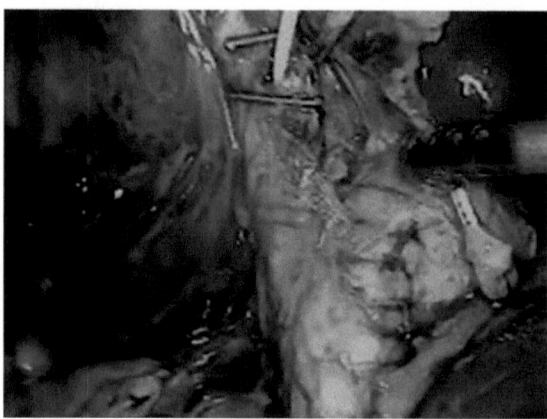

Figure 32 – Ideal choledochotomy

Tips and triks from senior surgeon:

1. Always perform intraoperative cholangiography in preoperative evidence (ultrasound) for gallbladder filled with numerous small gallstones, past episodes of jaundice, elevated alkaline phosphatase.

2. Perform longitudinal choledochotomy (1.5 cm) for diagnosed choledocholithiasis to revise laparoscopically the biliary tract and to extract the gallstones.

3. In case of doubt regarding patency of the biliary tract, insert Kerr drainage after the procedure.

6. Spilling of gallstones into the peritoneal cavity.

In the era of laparoscopic cholecystectomy accidental rupture of the wall of the gallbladder and spillage of gallstones into the peritoneal cavity is common. It happens in 20-40% of the cases. /10, 11/ Risk factors for injury to the gallbladder are: acute cholecystitis, pigmentary nature of stones, number of gallstones more than 15, lack of experience of the surgeon. Unfortunately gallstones spilled in the peritoneal cavity can cause a number of late complications, including life-threatening ones as: intra-abdominal abscesses, fistulas, intestinal obstruction. Most commonly concrements localize in the pocket of Morrison at the entrance of foramen Winslowi, in the space between the diaphragm and the liver, but may be found anywhere in the peritoneal cavity./10, 11, 35, 45, 47, 49/ Complications related to "lost" gallstones are usually manifested 12-15 months after the intervention. Diagnostic presentation is similar to pesentation of intra-abdominal abscesses, which are difficult to relate to surgery in the past. In CT examination radiopaque gallstones can sometimes be seen at the base of the abscess cavity. Figure 35

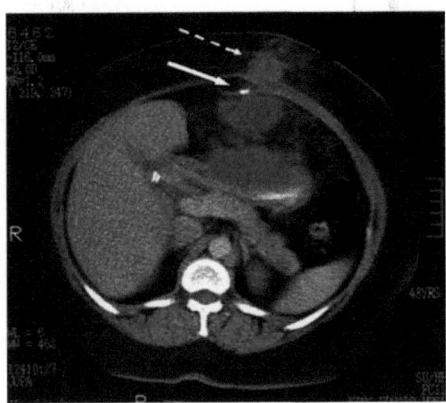

Figure 35 – Gallstones in the abscess cavity of the abdominal wall /52/

After S. Cheddie, L. Allopi, B. Singh: "Spilled,, Gallstones Causing Abdominal Wall Abscess. The Internet Journal of Surgery. 2012 Volume 28 Number 4.

The reason for abscess formation usually becomes clear during intervention for drainage of the collection when some or all scattered concretions are found. In our practice we had a patient who had to undergo three incisions of the anterior abdominal wall because of abscess 16 months after laparoscopic cholecystectomy. We have removed dozens of gallstones from the abscess cavity. Figure 36

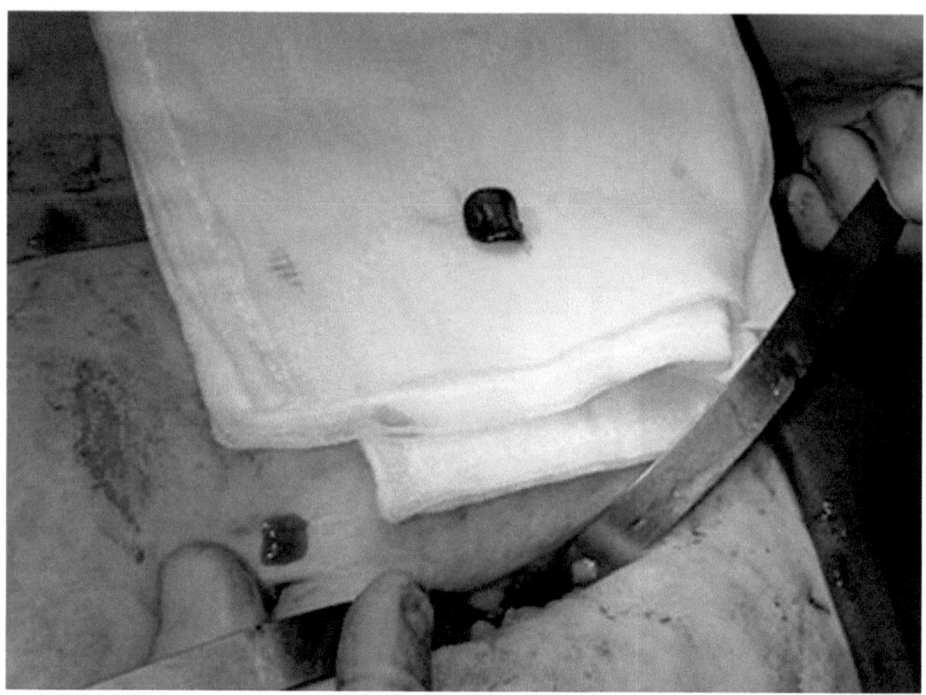

Figure 36 – Concretion from abdominal wall abscess

This complication can be prevented in of two steps. The first aims to prevent interference with the integrity of the gallbladder. In this aspect, the key factors are the use of atraumatic graspers when possible, and careful handling during monopolar coagulation when separating the bladder from the liver bed. The second step is to collect all gallstones that have dropped during surgery in an endobag (endoscopic bag) and remove them together with gallbladder. Figure 37

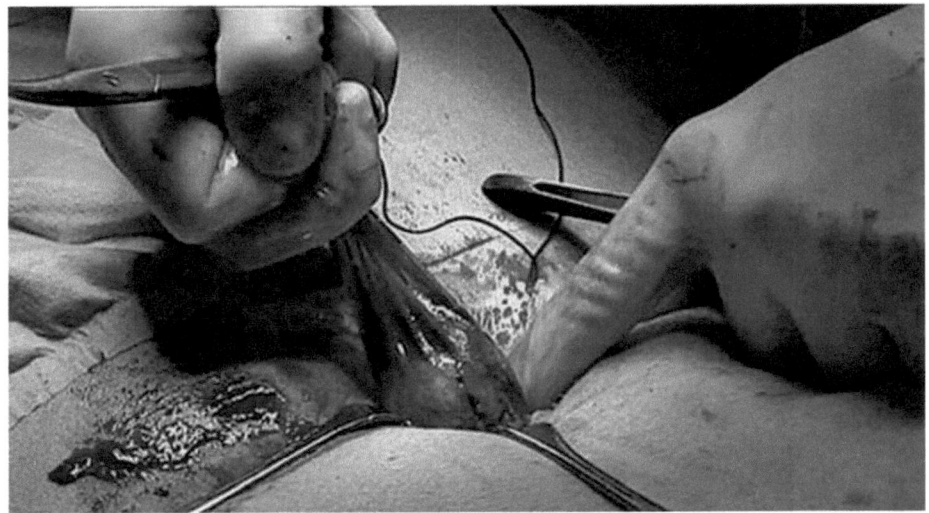

Figure 37

Tips and triks from senior surgeon:

1. In the case of spilling of gallstones from the gallbladder during surgery do not wait for the end of surgery. Collect them carefully and place them in Morrison's pocket . At the end of the procedure, you can easily find them and put them together with the gallbladder in the endobag.

2. When the diameter of spilled concretions is less than 7-8 mm, insert 10 mm aspiration cannula and aspirate the concretions. They are difficult to control regarding their localtion and collection.

3. Since in most cases the spilling of gallstones occurs in the very moment of removing the bladder through the periumbilical incision, always use endobag to remove it.

7. Suppuration of the surgical wound.

Inflammation of the surgical wound (periumbilical incision) is a complication that actually reduces the positive effect of minimum trauma in laparoscopic cholecystectomy. Albeit insignificant at first sight, it prolongs outpatient treatment and prevents early return to normal daily activities. In the second place surgical wound infection is a predisposing factor for the development of dehiscence of edges and formation of postoperative (incisional) hernia. Predisposing factors for surgical wound infection are general and local.

General factors include in the first place destructive forms of acute cholecystitis as an indication for laparoscopic cholecystectomy. The second place is taken by all the comorbidities, lowering the immunity of patients (diabetes mellitus, morbid obesity, immunodeficiencies). Local factors are the presence of a large amount of subcutaneous fat, trauma to the layers of the abdominal wall from rough manipulations with tools and retractrors, presence of subcutaneous hematoma. The microbiological agents most often isolated from the wound secretions are E.colli, Enterococcus and other pathogens which are usually isolated from the bile. Rarely the causes can be Staphylococcus aureus and Pseudomonas aeruginosa as typical representatives of nosocomial infection./51/

The path of spreading infection to the surgical wound is its mechanical contamination during removal of the gallbladder through the periumbilical incision. In nosocomial infections the pathway is through contaminated hands, tools, linens, etc. The clinical manifestation of the complication is similar to the one in postoperative infections in open surgery wounds. It is characterized by pain in wound region, swelling, redness, cloudy secretion from the wound edge, and general and local higher temperature. Diagnosis of this complication is relatively easy due to its superficial nature (develops in front of our eyes). Its treatment is not different from that in patients subjected to conventional surgery.

Prevention of wound infection

Prevention of wound infection is the true solution to this thorny problem. It consists of several steps. The first step is preoperative compensation and stabilization of common diseases interfering with immunity. Second is the prevention of penetration of pathogens in the surgical wound. This is done exclusively by means of the use of laparoscopic surgery bags for extraction , in which the removed gallbladder is placed prior to its removal from the peritoneal cavity. Third is the use of gentle atraumatic operative technique in shaping the periumbilical incision. Fourth is the use of antibiotics prophylaxis according to the standards of the specific method. Fifth is the use of antibacterial threads in closing the surgical wound and last, but not least in importance is the assessment whether to apply drainage to the surgical wound when indications are present .

Tips and triks from senior surgeons:

1. In cholecystectomy related to destructive inflammation of the gallbladder it is a must to use the endobag for its extraction.

2. In these cases drain the surgical wound with a simple pipe drain of a small diameter to prevent the formation of seroma.

3. Do not traumatize excessively the subcutaneous fat in increasing the fascial incision for the removal of the bladder.

8. Formation of postoperative /incisional/ hernia

Formation of postoperative /incisional/ hernia after laparoscopic cholecystectomy is another complication that compromises the short period of recovery after surgery. It is an immediate threat to the lives of patients through the possibility of incarceration and necrosis of the abdominal organs but also a disruptive factor significantly impairing the quality of life of patients without incarceration. The first report of the formation of postoperative hernia after laparoscopic cholecystectomy was done by Maio et al in 1991./36/

The incidence of the complication covers an average of 1.7% of the cases (0.3-5.4). /3, 8, 12, 15, 18, 24/

Postoperative hernias are localized mostly in the umbilical area, but there are reported cases of hernia in the epigastrium, the left and right hypochondrium. /15, 18, 24/

The only classification of this complication described in the literature divides hernias into early (dehiscence of the fascia and the peritoneum), late (dehiscence of the fascia with preserved integrity of the peritoneum) and specific (dehiscence of all layers of the abdominal wall).

Predisposing factors for this complication are divided into two main groups.

1. Patient factors - the availability of umbilical or paraumbilical hernia, obesity, size of gallstones in the gallbladder, diabetes, COPD, CKD, immunodeficiency, and infection of the surgical wound are identified as crucial in terms of increased risk of postoperative hernia.

2. Factors of the operational technique - diameter and type of trocar, closure of the fascial defect, the presence of a drain in the trocar opening, an extension of the fascial periumbilical incision are the most important predispositions to the formation of hernia.

The clinical presentation of the complication is associated with the emergence of pain in the affected area, swelling of various degrees, events of intestinal obstruction, strangulation or incarceration. When hernia content is presented by the omentum without intestinal loops, pain and discomfort are predominant. Treatment of postoperative hernia is in compliance with the general principles of surgical treatment of hernia. The prevention of this complication consists of the correction of the factors related to the patient, meticulous closure of fascial defects with single nonabsorbable sutures with atraumatic needle and prevention of operative wounds infection.

Tips and triks from senior surgeons:

1. *In cases of acute cholecystitis use endobag for the removal of the gallbladder.*
2. *Pay particular attention to closing the upper pole of the fascial incision. It usually remains "hidden" from the subcutaneous adipose tissue and its closure is uncertain.*
3. *When possible, perform total mini-laparatomy closure (of fascia and peritoneum) after removal of the gallbladder.*
4. *Use single interrupted suture with slowly absorbable stiches № 2.*

Literature

1. Belokonski E. „Complications in laparoscopic surgery„in „Laparoscopic surgery", Pogarliev T., 2008, Sofia, 15, AI"Prof.Marin Drinov" 266-278

2. Damjanov D, Lozanov R. „Laparoscopic surgery of the billiary tract",in in „Laparoscopic surgery", Pogarliev T., 2008, Sofia, 15, AI"Prof.Marin Drinov" 266-278

3. Alptekin H, Yilmaz H, Acar F, Kafali ME, Sahin M. Incisional hernia rate may increase afer single-port cholecystectomy. J Laparoendosc Adv Surg Tech A. 2012 Oct;22(8):731-7

4. Arshad M Malik, Abdul Aziz Laghari, Qasim Mallah, Fazila Hashmi, Ubaid Sheikh, and K Altaf Hussain Talpur. Extra-biliary complications during laparoscopic cholecystectomy: How serious is the problem? J Minim Access Surg. 2008 Jan-Mar;4(1): 5–8.

5. A. Shamiyeh, W. Wayand. Laparoscopic cholecystectomy:early and late complications and their treatment. Langenbecks Arch Surg (2004) 389:164–171

6. Bailey R.W., Gluck E.S. „Cholecystectomy" in „Managing complications of general surgery" in „Complications of Laparoscopic Surgery" 1995; Quality Medical Publishing. Inc. 77-124

7. Bulian DR, Trump L, Knuth J, Cerasani N, Heiss MM. Long-term results of transvaginal/transumbilical versus classical laparoscopic cholecystectomy--an analysis of 88 patients. Langenbecks Arch Surg. 2013 Apr;398(4):571-9

8. Bunting DM. Port-Site Hernia Following Laparoscopic Cholecystectomy Journal of the Society of Laparoendoscopic Surgeons. (2010)14:490–497

9. Burcharth J, Burgdorf S, Lolle I, Rosenberg J. Successful resuscitation afer carbon dioxide embolism during laparoscopy. Surg Laparosc Endosc Percutan Tech. 2012 Jun;22(3):e164-7.

10. Castellón Pavón CJ, Fernández Bermejo M, Morales Artero S, Del Amo Olea E. Subhepatic abscess as a late complication of missed intraperitoneal gallstone afer laparoscopic cholecystectomy. Gastroenterol Hepatol. 2004 Dec;27(10):568-72.

11. Castellón-Pavón CJ, Morales-Artero S, Martínez-Pozuelo A, Valderrábano-González S. Complications due to spilled gallstones and surgical clips lef in the abdomen during laparoscopic cholecystectomy. Cir Esp. 2008 Jul;84(1):3-9.

12. Coda A, Bossotti M, Ferri F, et al. Incisional hernia and fascial defect following laparoscopic surgery. Surg Laparosc Endosc Percutan Tech. 2000;10:34 – 38.

13. Connor S, Garden OJ. Bile duct injury in the era of laparoscopic cholecystectomy. Br J Surg. 2006;93(2):158–68.

14. Conzo G, Amato G, Angrisani L, Bardi U, Barone G, Belli G, et all. Surgical treatment of iatrogenic bile duct injuries following laparoscopic cholecystectomy: analysis of long-term results. Retrospective clinical study in 51 patients operated in the Campania region from 1991 to 2003.Chir Ital. 2005 Jul-Aug;57(4):417-24.

15. David Mark Bunting.Port-Site Hernia Following Laparoscopic Cholecystectomy. JSLS (2010)14:490–497

16. Delis S, Bakoyiannis A, Madariaga J, Bramis J, Tassopoulos N, Dervenis C. Laparoscopic cholecystectomy in cirrhotic patients: the value of MELD score and Child-Pugh classifcation in predicting outcome. Surg Endosc. 2010; 24 (2): 407–412.

17. Duca S, Bãlã O, Al-Hajjar N, Lancu C, Puia IC, Munteanu D, Graur F.Laparoscopic cholecystectomy: incidents and complications. A retrospective analysis of 9542 consecutive laparoscopic operations. HPB (Oxford). 2003; 5(3):152-8.

18. Dulskas A, Lunevičius R, Stanaitis J. A case report of incisional hernia through a 5 mm lateral port site following laparoscopic cholecystectomy. J Minim Access Surg. 2011 Jul;7(3):187-9

19. Eun Young Park, Ja-Young Kwon, Ki Jun Kim .Carbon Dioxide Embolism during Laparoscopic Surgery.Yonsei Med J. 2012 May 1; 53(3): 459–466.

20. Giger UF, Michel JM, Opitz I, T Inderbitzin D, Kocher T, Krähenbühl L; Risk factors for perioperative complications in patients undergoing laparoscopic cholecystectomy: analysis of 22,953 consecutive cases from the Swiss Association of Laparoscopic and Toracoscopic Surgery database.J Am Coll Surg. 2006 Nov;203(5):723-8. Epub 2006 Sep 20.

21. Hamad MA, Nada AA, Abdel-Atty MY, Kawashti AS. Major biliary complications in 2,714 cases of laparoscopic cholecystectomy without intraoperative cholangiography: a multicenter retrospective study. Surg Endosc. 2011 Dec;25(12):3747-51.

22. Hashizume M, Sugimachi K. Needle and trocar injury during laparoscopic surgery in Japan.Surg Endosc. 1997 Dec;11(12):1198-201.

23. Huang X, Feng Y, Huang Z. Complications of laparoscopic cholecystectomy in China: an analysis of 39,238 cases. Chin Med J (Engl). 1997 Sep;110(9):704-6.

24. Hussain A, Mahmood H, Singhal T, Balakrishnan S, Nicholls J, El-Hasani S. Long-term study of port-site incisional hernia afer laparoscopic procedures. JSLS 2009;13(3):346 –349.

25. Jablonska B, Lampe P. Iatrogenic bile duct injuries: Etiolog y, diagnosis and management. World J Gastroenterol. 2009;15(33):4097–104.

26. Jawad Ahmad, Kevin McElvanna,Lloyd McKie,Mark Taylor,Tom Diamond. Biliary complications during a decade of increased cholecystectomy rate. Ulster Med J. 2012 May; 81(2): 79–82.

27. Ji W, Li L-T, Chen X-R, Li J-S. Application of laparoscopic cholecystectomy in patients with cirrhotic portal hypertension. Hepatobiliary Pancreat Dis Int. 2004; 3 (2): 270–274.

28. Jurczak F. Laparoscopic cholecystectomy with transgastric gallbladder extraction. Bull Acad Natl Med. 2011 Nov;195(8):1887-97; discussion 1897-8.

29. Krähenbühl L, Sclabas G, Wente MN, Schäfer M, Schlumpf R, Büchler M W. Incidence, risk factors, and prevention of biliary tract injuries during laparoscopic cholecystectomy in Switzerland. World J Surg. 2001 Oct;25(10):1325-30.

30. Lau WY, Lai EC, Lau SH. Management of bile duct injury afer laparoscopic cholecystectomy: a review. ANZ J Surg. 2010;80((1-2)):75–81.

31. Leandros E, Albanopoulos K, Tsigris C, et al. Laparoscopic cholecystectomy in cirrhotic patients with symptomatic gallstone disease. ANZ J Surg. 2008; 78: 363–365.

32. Leunq E,Kumar P.Bilo-enteric fstula (BEF) at laparoscopic cholecystectomy: Review of ten year's experience.,Te Surgeon,Volume 8, Issue 2 , Pages 67-70, April 2010

33. Li F, Frilling A, Nadalin S, Paul A, Malago M, Broelsch CE. Management of concomitant hepatic artery injury in patients with iatrogenic major bile duct injury afer laparoscopic cholecystectomy. Br J Surg. 2008;95(4):460–5.

35. Maempel J, Darmanin G, Paice A, Uzkalnis A. An unusual „hernia": losing a stone is not always a good thing! BMJ Case Rep. 2009;2009. pii: bcr12.2008.132

36. Maio A, Ruchman RB. CT diagnosis of postlaparoscopic hernia. J Comput Assist Tomogr. 1991 Nov-Dec;15(6):1054 –1055.

37. Mala S.Prevention of common bile duct injuries in laparoscopic cholecystectomy.World J Lap Surg 2012;5(1)27-32

38. Massarweh NN, Flum DR: Role of intraoperative cholangiography in avoiding bile duct injury. J Am Coll Surg 204:656–664,2007.

39. Mrksić MB, Farkas E, Cabaf Z, Komlos A, Sarac M. Complications in laparoscopic cholecystectomy. Med Pregl. 1999 Jun-Aug;52(6-8):253-7.

40. Nera Agabiti, Massimo Stafoggia Marina Davoli, Danilo Fusco, Anna Patrizia Barone, Carlo Alberto Perucci. Tirty-day complications afer laparoscopic or open cholecystectomy: a population-based cohort study in Italy. BMJ Open. 2013; 3(2): e001943.

41. Norman Oneil Machado Laparoscopic Cholecystectomy in Cirrhotics JSLS. 2012 Jul-Sep; 16(3): 392–400.

42. Nuzzo G, Giuliante F, Giovannini I, et al: Advantages of multidisciplinary management of bile duct injuries occurring during cholecystectomy. Am J Surg 195:763–769, 2008.

43. Pavlidis TE, Symeonidis NG, Psarras K, et al. Laparoscopic cholecystectomy in patients with cirrhosis of the liver and symptomatic cholelithiasis. JSLS. 2009; 13: 342–345

44. Parmeggiani D, Cimmino G, Cerbone D, Avenia N, Ruggero R, Gubitosi A, Docimo G, Mordente S, Misso C, Parmeggiani U. Biliary tract injuries during laparoscopic cholecystectomy: three case reports and literature review. G Chir. 2010 Jan-Feb;31(1-2):16-9.

45. Patterson EJ, Nagy AG. Don't cry over spilled stones? Complications of gallstones spilled during laparoscopic cholecystectomy: case report and literature review. Can J Surg. 1997 Aug;40(4):300-4.

46. Pekolj J, Alvarez FA, Palavecino M, Sánchez Clariá R, Mazza O, de Santibañes E. Intraoperative Management and Repair of Bile Duct Injuries Sustained during 10,123 Laparoscopic Cholecystectomies in a High-Volume Referral Center. J Am Coll Surg. 2013 May;216(5):894-901

47. Rammohan A, Srinivasan U P, Jeswanth S, Ravichandran P. Infammatory pseudotumour secondary to spilled intra-abdominal gallstones. Int J Surg Case Rep. 2012;3(7):305-7. doi: 10.1016/j. ijscr.2012.03.013. Epub 2012 Mar 23.

48. Rapicetta Cristian, Paci Massimiliano, Ricchetti Tommaso,Tenconi Sara, Biolchini Federico, Belluzzi Emilio, and Sgarbi Giorgio Massive right hemothorax as the source of hemorrhagic shock afer laparoscopic cholecystectomy - case report of a rare intraoperative complication Patient Saf Surg. 2011; 5: 12.

49. Riaz N, Khurshaidi N, Abdullah SS. Complications of spilled gallstones during laparoscopic cholecystectomy: case series with review of literature. J Coll Physicians Surg Pak. 2007 Dec;17(12):758-60.

50. Rooh-ul-Muqim,Qutab-e-Alam   Jan,Mohammad   Zarin,Mehmud Aurangziab,Aziz Wazir.,,Complications of laparoscopic cholecystectomy,,,World Journal of Laparoscopic Surgery,Jan-April 2008;1(1):1-5

51. Romy S, Eisenring MC, Bettschart V, et al. Laparoscope use and surgical site infections in digestive surgery. Ann Surg 2008;247:627–32.

52. S. Cheddie, L. Allopi , B. Singh : „Spilled" Gallstones Causing Abdominal Wall Abscess. Te Internet Journal of Surgery. 2012 Volume 28 Number 4.

53. Sanjeev Kumar Sareen,,, Cholecystoduodenal Fistula is not the Contraindication for Laparoscopic Surgery,,, World Journal of Laparoscopic Surgery, January-April 2011;4(1):41-46

54. Sasmal PK, Tantia O, Jain M, Khanna S, Sen B. Primary access-related complications in laparoscopic cholecystectomy via the closed technique: experience

of a single surgical team over more than 15 years. Surg Endosc. 2009 Nov;23(11):2407-15

55. Shaikh AR, Muneer A. Laparoscopic cholecystectomy in cirrhotic patients. JSLS. 2009; 13: 592–596.

56. Schif J, Misra M, Rendon G, Rothschild J, Schwaitzberg S. Laparoscopic cholecystectomy in cirrhotic patients. Surg Endosc. 2005; 19 (9): 1278–1281.

57. Singh R, Kaushik R, Sharma R, Attri AK. Non-biliary mishaps during laparoscopic cholecystectomy. Indian J Gastroenterol. 2004 Mar-Apr;23(2):47-9.

58. Strasberg SM, Brunt LM. Rationale and Use of the Critical View of Safety in Laparoscopic Cholecystectomy. J Am Coll Surg. 2010;211(1):132–8.

59. Tomas Kjeld, Egon G Hansen, Nana G Holler,3 Henrik Rottensten, Ole Hyldegaard, and Eric C Jansen. Resuscitation by hyperbaric exposure from a venous gas emboli following laparoscopic surgery. Scand J Trauma Resusc Emerg Med. 2012; 20: 51.

60. Tomson BN, Parks RW, Madhavan KK, Wigmore SJ, Garden OJ. Early specialist repair of biliary injury. Br J Surg. 2006;93(2):216–20.

61. Tonouchi H, Ohmori Y, Kobayashi M, Kusonoki M. Trocar site hernia. Arch Surg. 2004;139:1248 –1256.

62. Triantafyllidis I, Nikoloudis N, Sapidis N, Chrissidou M, Kalaitsidou I, Chrissidis T. Complications of laparoscopic cholecystectomy: our experience in a district general hospital.Surg Laparosc Endosc Percutan Tech. 2009 Dec;19(6):449-58.

63. Walsh RM, Henderson JM, Vogt DP, et al: Long-term outcome of biliary reconstruction for bile duct injuries from laparoscopic cholecystectomies. Surgery 142:450–456, 2007.

64. Way LW, Stewart L, Gantert W, et al: Causes and prevention of laparoscopic bile duct injuries: Analysis of 252 cases from a human factors and cognitive psychology perspective. Ann Surg 237:460– 469, 2003.

65. Yamakawa T, Zhang T, Midorikawa Y, Ishiyama J, Takahashi K, Sugiyama Y. A case of cystic duct drainage into the lef intrahepatic duct and the importance of laparoscopic fundus-frst cholecystectomy for prevention of bile duct injury. J Laparoendosc Adv Surg Tech A. 2007 Oct;17(5):662-5.

66. Yavuz Selim Sari, Vahit Tunali, Kamer Tomaoglu, Binnur Karagöz, Ayhan Güneyİİbrahim KaragöZ .Can bile duct injuries be prevented? „A new technique in laparoscopic cholecystectomy" BMC Surg. 2005; 5: 14.

67. Yetkin G, Uludag M, Oba S, et al. Laparoscopic cholecystectomy in elderly patients. JSLS 2009;13:587–91.

68. Yi F, Jin WS, Xiang DB, Sun GY, Huaguo D. Complications of laparoscopic cholecystectomy and its prevention: a review and experience of 400 cases. Hepatogastroenterology. 2012 Jan-Feb;59(113):47-50

69. Zha Y, Chen XR, Luo D, Jin Y. Te prevention of major bile duct injures in laparoscopic cholecystectomy: the experience with 13,000 patients in a single center. Surg Laparosc Endosc Percutan Tech. 2010 Dec;20(6):378-83.

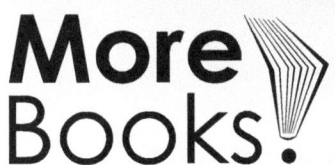
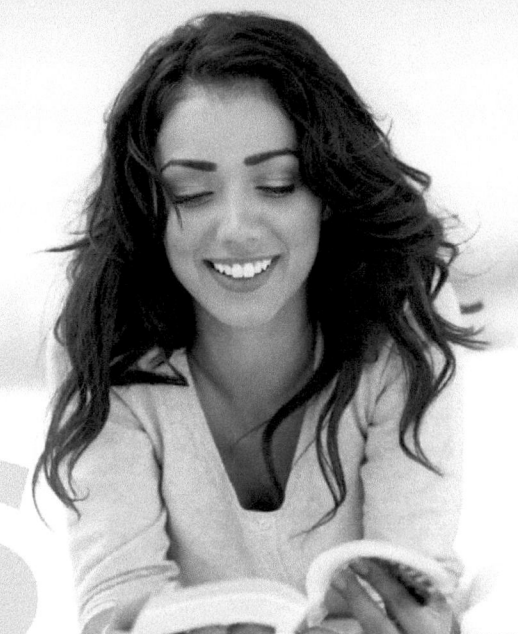
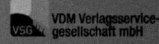

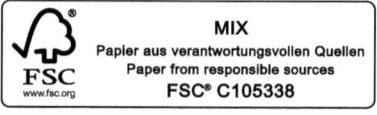